HOW TO

Look & Feel

FABULOUS

AFTER

50

Carime Muvdi

Simple Health Tips to Eat Better
Have More Energy, Avoid Sugar Cravings
and Lose Weight In The Process

CARIME MUVDI

Website: howtolookandfeelfabulousafter50.com
Email: contact@howtolookandfeelfabulousafter50.com
Facebook: www.facebook.com/HowtoLookandFeelFabulousAfter50
Instagram: www.instagram.com/carimemuvdi
Twitter: www.twitter.com/lmuvdi

DEDICATION

I want to dedicate this book to all the "super women" in the world that want to do a change in their lifestyle to look and feel fabulous after 50. All these women who are daughters, mothers, mothers and fathers, professionals, head of households, workers, divas, lovers, etc.

ENJOY LIFE!

CONTENTS

INTRODUCTION

When you reach the magic number of 50, it is when you realize your body is starting to change: the way you look, the way you feel, your memory, your motivation, white hairs, hair loss, energy, libido, your relationships, everything.

In this book, I will show you how, by following my advice, you will feel great, look amazing, have more energy, avoid sugar cravings, lose weight in the process and live a happy and fulfilling life.

It is not a fad diet, that just works for a few months, it is not a magic pill or beauty cream that will not make you age, it is not a detox tea or a plastic surgeon that will make you look great. It is what you do on a daily basis that will make you look and feel fabulous after 50. It is not a diet; it is a lifestyle. Lifestyle choices that can exert significant control over your biological age!

I consider myself a student who is always learning to be able to transmit what I know and help other people. I am an AFAA certified Personal Trainer, Aerobic Instructor, Spinning instructor, Holistic

Nutritionist, Health Coach and Raw Vegan Chef. I worked as an aerobics instructor and personal trainer in Colombia and the U.S.A for 20 years. I had a TV show about Fitness, and I have given talks about nutrition. My Luzkis protein bars have been acclaimed in Bazaar Arabia and have helped clients achieve their goals through proper nutrition and lifestyle advice.

Many women of all ages who struggle with health and weight issues, bad eating habits, low self-esteem and no motivation have experienced great success by implementing the tips and advice in this helpful "How to guide."

The best thing about this book is that is easy to read and follow. It will not take too much of your time to read it, but it will make a difference in the way you feel and look.

I promise that if you follow my advice, you will see results; you will feel more energetic, look and feel better, and the most important, you will love yourself and make yourself happy.

Do not be the woman who is jealous of other women who look, feel great and confident about themselves. Take action today and be that woman that you would like to be. Start loving yourself by taking care of your body and your spirit. Start doing what you like. We as women always take care of our children, husbands, boyfriends, parents, friends but we never have the time for ourselves. Make the time; love yourself so you can age gracefully by being in shape, healthy and happy.

The nutrition, fitness, and lifestyle tips you are about to read have been proven to help avoid disease, increase energy, avoid sugar cravings, lose weight and live a happier and more productive life after 50.

CHAPTER 1
NUTRITION

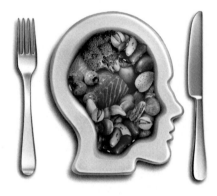

Nutrition is the process of taking in food and using it for growth, metabolism and repair. It is the act of nourishing or being nourished. We have the Primary Foods and the Secondary Foods. Primary Foods are all those things that feed us beyond our plate: our spirituality, jobs, relationships, recreational and physical activities. As the Institute for Integrative Nutrition teaches, "When primary food is balanced and satiated, your life feeds you, making what you actually eat secondary." (Rosenthal)

Secondary foods are what we actually eat. This is the difference between primary and secondary foods. You need both to feel great!!! Whenever we are not feeling well, or something is not feeling right, it could be an imbalance of either your primary or secondary foods.

We will start by the secondary foods. What I do as a holistic nutritionist is give guidance and inspiration to help women shift their behavior to healthier habits by making step-by-step changes to their diet and lifestyle. I give advice on weight management, the meaning of sugar cravings and how to avoid it, how to increase energy by eating the right foods, how to avoid disease by making right food choices, how to avoid gaining weight after menopause, how to eat after cancer, etc.

There are too many fad diets right now that promise you to lose weight. I am sure we have all tried one of them. Have they worked for you in the long run? Every person is unique and what works for me may not work for you. The key to health is to understand each person's individual needs, rather than following predetermined rules. It is not the same if you are an active person, if you are training for a marathon, if you are sedentary, just had a baby, want to be a vegetarian, are going through cancer, have diabetes or reactive hypoglycemia, etc.

I have seen that having good relationships – family, friends, a fulfilling career, an exercise routine and a spiritual practice – are even more important to health than any kind of diet. We will talk about this, Primary Foods, in another chapter.

I am going to talk first about how to keep healthy and how to lose weight and feel great in the process.

Nowadays, most of the foods that are sold in supermarkets and fast food restaurants are processed. These foods are packaged in beautiful colorful boxes such as cereals, frozen foods, candies, etc. All this processed foods have additives and chemicals to make them have a long shelf life. In the list of ingredients we find words that are hard to pronounce and we do not even know where these ingredients come from. A lot of added sugars are added to the processed foods to make them taste good. All of these additives and chemicals produce side effects such as headaches, cancer, Alzheimer, diabetes, high blood pressure, heart problems, obesity, among others.

The first thing we have to learn is to read the ingredients found in the foods we buy and not let us get influenced by deceiving Marketing "tactics" such as low fat, low sugar, low calories. Many of these " low fat products" are loaded with sugar to make them taste good.

Sugar, a form of carbohydrate, is quickly available to be converted to energy, but if sugar calories are not used as energy shortly after they are consumed, they are converted into stored body fat by a process known as lipogenesis.

According to nutritionist Dr. Jonny Bowden, fructose is converted to fat more quickly than any other type of sugar. Fructose is the sugar found in fruit, often extracted and processed into the ubiquitous high-fructose corn syrup. Fruit, however, contains relatively low levels of fructose when compared to foods with processed sugar. In addition, fruit are whole foods that have fiber and nutrients. Therefore, fruit does not need to be eliminated from the diet, although those who have problems with weight gain or insulin resistance may want to limit their fruit consumption. (Bowden)

We have to avoid consuming high-fructose corn syrup and sugar. These refined sugars are added to many processed foods. They do not contain any vitamins, proteins or fiber. These are "empty calories" that can cause blood sugar levels to spike, which in turn causes insulin levels to rise. Insulin is a hormone released by the body that helps regulate blood sugar levels. If sugar is not quickly used for energy, insulin removes it from the blood, and it is then converted into triglycerides in the liver. These triglycerides can then be stored as body fat. (Mcnight, "Does Sugar Turn Into Fat?")

List of Controversial ingredients to avoid:

1. Artificial Sweeteners

Artificial sweeteners such as Saccharin (Sweet'N Low), Aspartame (Equal), and Sucralose (Splenda) are man made toxic chemicals that your body was never intended to use. They are made to give the sweet taste of sugar but without the calories.

Saccharin was discovered accidentally while researching for Toluene derivatives. Toluene is a liquid produced during the process of making gas from crude oil and is registered as a hazardous chemical. Sucralose was discovered while researching for new insecticides. It contains a lot of chlorine. Aspartame is metabolized and breaks down into things such as methanol, which can cause definite health problems. (Tomberlin)

These artificial sweeteners can produce anxiety, headaches, nausea, depression, allergic reactions, obesity and many other things that are detrimental to our health.

You may ask yourself why obesity if they do not have calories? According to a study by Purdue University, artificial sweeteners interrupt the natural ability to regulate the amount of calories consumed based in the sweetness of the food. This means that when you consume diet sodas or anything sweetened with artificial sweeteners, you are more predisposed to eat more because your body is being deceived that is eating sugar and makes you crave for more sugar. I do not understand how people, who call themselves "fitness experts" or "Nutritionists", recommend people to eat protein bars or whey protein sweetened with artificial sweeteners such as sucralose.

There are other healthy alternatives to sweeten your food such as with dates, maple syrup, honey or coconut sugar and if you can not have sugar because of health issues such as Diabetes or you are trying to lose weight you can sweeten your foods or beverages with Stevia. I recommend the liquid Stevia that does not contain preservatives or stabilizers.

2. Refined sugars

In the United States, people are consuming between 130 to 160 pounds of sugar per year. In other words people are consuming ½ to 1 cup of sugar per day and they do not even know where it comes from. To make processed foods and beverages taste good they are loaded with sugar so consumers get addicted to them. Sugar is found in canned soups, ketchup, juices, teas, processed cereal, etc. That is why it is so important to READ LABELS:

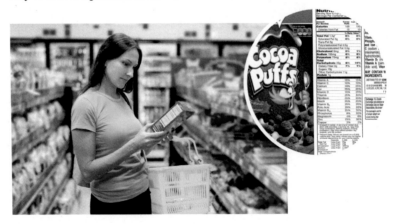

For every 4 grams of sugar there is 1 tablespoon of sugar, so you divide the total amount of grams by 4 to find out how many tablespoons of sugar your serving has. Also it says that the amounts they are giving you is according to ¾ cup, which means you have to do the math if you serve yourself 1 cup. So if it contains 10 grams of sugar in ¾ cup then you have 2.5 tablespoons of sugar, but most likely is that you are going to have at least a full cup serving so you will have to add 2.5 more grams of sugars to the equation (0.25 x 10 grams) which will be equal to .62 tablespoon more of sugar. Confusing? Yes and that is what big food manufacturers do to make it look like if their products have less sugar. This is a typical example when you buy a juice or tea. The label usually tells you the amount of sugar for 8 ounces when they usually are 16 ounces (in this case you will have to multiply the amounts by 2). No wonder diabetes is becoming an epidemic.

It is a proven fact that sugar creates addiction. There are studies that have proven that sugar creates even more addiction than cocaine. (Ahmed, et al)

I have had clients who come to me with sugar cravings and soda addiction. I usually recommend them adding vegetable juices, fruits and green tea to their diet. The natural sugars found in the vegetable juices and fruits stop them from craving processed sugar and the caffeine found in the green tea stops the craving for the caffeine found in sodas.

3. MSG - Monosodium Glutamate

This is a very common additive that is added to make processed foods tastier. It is found in canned vegetables, frozen foods, fast foods and canned soups. MSG produces headaches, digestive issues, rashes, dizziness, heart and respiratory problems. ("MSG Side Effects") (Zeratsky)

4. Artificial Colors

Artificial colors such as blue, red, yellow and green are very common in juices, cereals and yoghurts and usually the ones that are used are not natural. All these artificial colors are used by the big food industry manufacturers to make processed foods more appealing and visually attractive. Most of these artificial colors are made with arsenic and lead and they are approved by the FDA as safe. This is due to the fact that the big food industries in the US have a lot of political power. Artificial colors can cause allergic reactions and hyperactivity in children with ADD. (Mcnight, "The Side Effects of Artificial Food Coloring")

5. Butylated Hydroxyanisole (BHA) and Butylated Hydroxytoluene (BHT)

These are additives used by the food industry to prevent oils from becoming rancid. There have been studies that BHA has caused stomach cancer in rats. ("Two Preservatives to Avoid?")

6. Sodium Nitrate and Nitrates

They are preservatives that are added to processed meats, such as ham and sausages, to increase the red color and flavors. These chemicals have been linked to cancer. They also cause headaches, vomiting, nausea and dizziness. If you love ham or turkey you can find them without these chemicals in health food stores and supermarkets or just cook an organic turkey and slice it.

I hope I am not boring you with all these hard to pronounce names, but it is very important that you know when you read your labels what to avoid. There was even a girl who told me in one of my lectures that she wrote them all down and use to take the list with her when she went to buy her groceries.

Ok so lets keep on. A few more:

7. Olestra (Olean)

It is synthetic oil that is also used in processed foods. It is not absorbed by the digestive tract. Olestra does not allow vitamins and minerals to get absorbed by the body.

8. Brominated Vegetable Oil

This additive when consumed is stored in the body as fat. It interferes with conception and can cause birth defects. Brominated Vegetable oil has been forbidden in 100 countries.

9. Hydrogenated Vegetable Oil

Known as Trans fats or trans-fatty acids. According to Mayo Clinic, trans fats are the worst type of fat you can eat. They increase your LDL (bad) cholesterol and lowers you HDL (good) cholesterol. A high LDL cholesterol level in combination with a low HDL cholesterol level increases your risk of heart disease, the leading killer of men and women.

Trans fats are used to prolong shelf life so it is found in a variety of food products, including: baked goods, cakes, cookies, pie crust, and crackers that contain shortening, which is usually made from partially hydrogenated vegetable oil. Ready- made frosting is another source of trans fat. Snacks such as Potatoes, corn, tortilla chips often contain trans fat. We even think we are eating a healthy snack when we eat popcorn, but many types that are packaged or microwavable use trans fats.

Fried foods – foods that require deep-frying such as French fries, doughnuts, and fried chicken – can contain trans fat from the oil used in the cooking process. Refrigerator Dough Products such as canned biscuits, frozen pizza crust and cinnamon rolls, creamers and margarines, non-dairy coffee creamer and stick margarine also may contain partially hydrogenated vegetable oils.

So now you ask yourself why are we getting sick? Why so many people have to take medicine to lower their cholesterol?

Reading food labels: In the United States, if a food has less than 0.5 grams of trans fat in a serving, the food label can read 0 grams trans fat. This hidden trans fat can add up specially if you eat several foods containing less than 0.5 grams a serving and this really adds up if you have been eating this since you were a child. It is important that when you read the food label for trans fat, check the food's ingredient list for partially hydrogenated vegetable oil, which indicates that the food contains some trans fat, even if the amount is below 0.5 grams.

So, you may ask yourself, what kind of fat can I use?

Monounsaturated fats which are the good fats found in olive oil, avocadoes and nuts.

This book-guide is marketed to women after 40 but everybody should read it. It is important to learn how to read labels. Know what you are eating to avoid eating foods that contain detrimental chemicals to your health that will cause disease and drug dependence.

10. Pesticides

Every year more than 2 billion pounds of pesticides are added to our food. This amounts to 10 pounds per person, scary? Pesticides can cause a variety of adverse health effects, ranging from simple irritation of the skin and eyes to more severe effects such as affecting the nervous system, mimicking hormones causing reproductive problems, and also causing cancer.

Then we ask ourselves why is there so much cancer?

Many clients tell me that is expensive to buy organic and I ask them what is more expensive to buy organic or being sick, paying high doctor's fees and hospital bills and not being able to work or enjoy life? Isn't it better just to save on other things such as $4.95 latte at the corner coffee shop or buying an expensive designer bag?

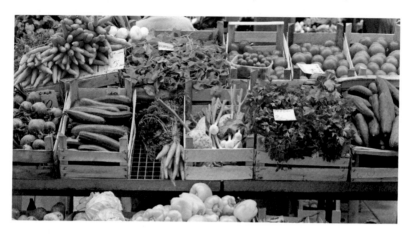

THE DIRTY DOZEN

Fruits and veggies with **the most pesticides are:**

Apples
Peaches
Nectarines
Strawberries
Grapes
Celery
Spinach
Sweet Bell Peppers
Cucumbers
Cherry Tomatoes
Snap Peas
Potatoes

The dirty dozen plus includes:
Hot Peppers
Kale/Collard Greens

THE CLEAN 15

Fruits and veggies with **the least pesticides are:**

Avocados
Sweet Corn
Pineapples
Cabbage
Sweet Peas (frozen)
Onion
Asparagus
Mangos
Papayas
Kiwis
Eggplant
Grapefruit
Cantaloupe
Cauliflower
Sweet Potatoes

So, if it works within your budget, it is recommendable to buy organic whenever possible, and if you can not get organic or if it is not in your budget, I would recommend to buy fruits and vegetables from the Clean 15 list instead. (Pou)

You may ask is it not safe just to wash the produce or peel them?
A study done at the Connecticut Agricultural Experiment Station confirms that washing is only partially effective. There is also the issue of systemic pesticides: these are chemicals designed to be absorbed by plants to kill any bugs that eat them. These poisons are inside the produce itself and will not be affected by washing.

The best practice when cleaning produce is:

- Discard the outer layer of leafy vegetables.
- Wash any produce you serve in running water, not a bath, especially if it is conventionally grown.
- Rub soft skin produce as you go.
- Scrub and /or peel produce that can take it.
- Never use dish soap or other products not intended for food.
- If you want to use a non-produce wash, look for one made with no-toxic ingredients that have been found to be effective. Otherwise you are wasting money and may be adding unwanted residue to your produce.

For me, the best way to clean my produce is by mixing vinegar and water at a 1-3 ratio. I soak them in my kitchen sink; this acidic blend kills all the bacteria such as E. coli and also it prevents them from molding within a few days of purchasing them. Then I scrub them with a brush and rinse them under running water.

When shopping, choose unbruised an undamaged produce. You should always wash oranges, pineapples, squash, melons and other produce with inedible rinds. Cutting or peeling the produce will transfer contaminants to the edible flesh. Another advice is not to buy packaged cut fruits or veggies. Besides being more expensive, once they are cut, they start losing their nutrients and they are not necessarily cleaner. The more a food item is handled and processed, the more likely it is that the item will come into contact with germs.

11. Genetically Modified Organism – GMOs

GMOs are living organism whose genetic material has been artificially manipulated in a laboratory through genetic engineering. This new science creates an unstable combination of plants, animal, bacteria and viral genes that do not occur in nature or through traditional crossbreeding methods. ("The History of Genetically Modified Foods")

Despite Biotech industry promises, none of the GMO traits currently on the market offer increased yield, enhanced nutrition or any other consumer benefit. A growing body of evidence connects GMOs with health problems, such as organ damage, gastrointestinal and immune system disorders, accelerated aging and infertility. Numerous health problems increased after GMOs were introduced in 1996. The percentage of Americans with three or more chronic illnesses jumped from 7% to 13 % in just 9 years; food allergies skyrocketed and disorders such as autism, reproductive disorders, and other disorders are on the rise. ("Health Risks")

The American Public Health Association and American Nurses Association are among many medical groups that condemn the use of GM bovine growth hormone, because the milk from treated cows has more of the hormone IGF-1 (insulin-like growth factor1), which is linked to cancer. (Group, "8 Shocking Facts about Bovine Growth Hormone")

That is why I do not drink milk, and I drink non-dairy alternative such as almond, cashew or coconut milk that I do myself. But if you really like milk, it is important to drink organic milk without these added hormones that will mess your metabolism. If you buy almond, cashew, hemp or coconut milk make sure they do not contain carrageenan. "This ingredient is the other big problem with many store-bought non-dairy milks. Carrageenan comes from red algae, and it is added to nut milks to stabilize and thicken them. Not only is carrageenan indigestible to the human stomach, it is also a known carcinogen". Bottom line do not buy any products with carrageenan. (Gioffre)

Many people in the Fitness industry recommend high doses of whey protein or protein bars with whey, which contain bovine growth hormone and are sweetened with sucralose. If you are going to use these supplements make sure you get them without sucralose, sweetened with Stevia and without Bovine Growth Hormone. There are two brands that I recommend of whey protein derived from grass fed cows, not treated with rBGH or Antibiotics and without sucralose, Bluebonnet and Jay Robb are both good brands. Both taste very good, do not contain GMOs and are sweetened with Stevia. They contain 25 grams of protein per serving and 0 grams of sugar.

GMOs are banned in most developed nations such as Japan, Australia and all of the countries in the European Union. There are significant restrictions or outright bans on the production and sale of GMOs. Sadly in the US, the government has approved GMOs based on studies conducted by the same corporations that produce them and profit from their sale. In the US, GMOs are in as much as 80% of conventional processed foods. (www.nongmoproject.org)

So, you may ask yourself what can I eat? It is worth it to be an educated consumer, especially if we are talking about our health and the health of our loved ones. Avoid processed foods!!! If your body is toxic your metabolism will not workout well. That is why today more than ever we have so many cases of diabetes, obesity, high blood pressure, heart problems, and cancer.

Shall we eat meat or chicken? Personally, I stopped eating red meat a long time ago because I noticed that every time I ate red meat I would sweat the whole night, especially in the area of my neck and face. Since I stopped eating red meat, I have not felt that anymore. I think it makes a big difference especially during menopause. Also, red meat is too slow to digest and makes me lethargic. You have to know your body and learn what works for you. If you want to avoid night sweats and not being able to sleep after 50, I would recommend not eating red meats.

Working out, doing a sport you love and yoga also helps. One study found that women who engaged in regular physical activity had fewer and less severe night sweats.

Chicken? They are loaded with hormones and antibiotics, which are harmful. If you feel the need to eat chicken or meat it would be wise to choose organic chickens and beef.

Personally, I have become a pescetarian. A pescetarian, means been a vegetarian while still including seafood in your diet. Cutting out red meat, pork, poultry, etc, from his or her diet like a vegetarian. (Spencer)

A pescetarian diet reduces your risk for heart disease and other cardiovascular diseases, stroke, osteoporosis, obesity, diabetes, arthritis, high blood pressure and some types of cancer. According to the Yale College Vegetarian society, 80% of cancers cases are preventable through healthy diets that contain low amounts of fats and oils and high amounts of fiber. (Hamblin)(Spencer)

Meat is often covered in pesticides and chemicals that are harmful, and after extended consumption, can be very dangerous, to humans. Every bite of a beef/pork hotdog contains seven cancer-causing pesticides. According to David Steinman's "Living Healthy in a Toxic World": The primary source of nuclear radiation contamination in humans is from beef and dairy products.

Also, I believe in no animal cruelty. The poor cows, pigs and chickens are being bred for murder in slaughterhouses. They are brought up in terrible conditions, packed into crates so crowded that they can hardly move. Chickens are kept also in crowded conditions in big warehouses. The chickens peck at each other, so their beaks are removed to prevent them from doing this. This is done without painkillers. They are injected with growth hormones so their breasts become so heavy that they sometimes can not even stand.

Hogs and cows are also treated terribly. They are hung upside down, still alive and taken down a belt to have their throats slit or beheaded by a machine. Many times the animal is not dead immediately, because their throat had only been nicked as they get hacked into pieces or boiled alive. (Spencer)

> " If slaughterhouses had glass walls,
> everyone would be a vegetarian. "
>
> – Paul McCartney

I recommend eating wild caught fish. It is digested much quicker than red meat. The Omega- 3 fatty acids, DHA and EPA that are present in seafood and fish are necessary in the diet of human beings.

Why wild fish and not farmed fish? We have to be informed consumers. Farmed fish is detrimental to your health!!! Farmed-fish are grown in overcrowded conditions, so they are given antibiotics to stave off disease that result from crowded conditions and also treated with pesticides to combat sea lice. Studies done by the Environmental Working Group, along with studies done in Canada, Ireland and the UK, have found that cancer – causing polychlorinated biphenyls (PCBs) exist in farm-raised salmon at 16 times the rate of wild salmon. Researchers have also found high levels of polybrominated diphenyl (PBDE) in farmed-raised fish, which are endocrine disruptors that are thought to contribute to cancer. ("PCBs in Farmed Salmon")

To add a pink color to farm raised salmon Canthaxanthin, a synthetic pigment is used. Studies have found that this chemical can affect pigments in the retina of the eye. This chemical is banned in many countries such as the UK. Farmed-Fish are also given growth hormones so they grow faster. (HGH) can increase the risk of diabetes and contribute to the growth of cancerous tumors, beside increasing your cholesterol levels, producing joint pain, edema, carpal tunnel syndrome and numbness and tingling of the skin. ("Changes in Sperm Parameters")

Fish farms do not combat overfishing; they contribute to it because some fish like salmon are carnivores. It takes about 2 ½ to 4 pounds of other fish to create the salmon chow needed to produce 1 pound of farm-raised salmon, so this creates overfishing of wild sardines, anchovies, mackerel, and other fish, which upsets the natural ecosystems.

This information should be enough to convince you to stay away from farm- fish and before you order fish at a restaurant or buy it in the supermarket make sure it is wild fish. Do not damage your health or contribute to the business of farmed-fish, which damages the ecosystem.

So, after reading about all these chemicals found in processed foods, pesticides, farm-fish, hormones, antibiotics and the inhumane conditions in which chickens, cows and hogs are raised you may ask yourself SO WHAT DO I EAT?

In America, most of us are accustomed to building our dinner plates around meat, eating processed foods because it does not take time to prepare and is convenient, giving our children sugar loaded cereals for breakfast, eating on the go or at fast food restaurants. If you want to exert control over your biological age and age well you will have to start making changes to the way you eat, exercise, sleep as well as to how you deal with the big and small stressors of life. Start by doing small changes to your eating habits and lifestyle. What is important is the long-term accumulation of small decisions and daily actions and not some dramatic "this is it or final answer" that has the best chance of leading to a healthy and happy life.

Stop Thinking About How Many Calories!

All calories are not created equal. With calories, as with diamonds, it is the quality that matters most. It is not the same 100 calories from an organic apple than 100 calories from a mini Snickers. Crap is crap no matter how many calories are involved. Calories from nutrient rich foods versus calories from processed or refined carbs will have different effects in your body. When we eat healthy, nutrient-rich foods, we keep our blood sugar levels stable, we do not get hungry all the time, we minimize cravings. Nutrient-poor foods will have the opposite effect, wreaking hormonal havoc, spiking insulin, setting off cravings, dulling satiety signals and encourage overeating. So, if you really do not want to gain weight and feel good YOU HAVE TO STOP EATING PROCCESED FOODS!!! It is simple. Trade hunger, calorie counting, for filling nutrient-dense, organic, local produce, pasture-raised meats (if you eat red meat) and wild fish. Eat them until you feel satisfied. When you eat good foods, your body will tell you when you have had enough. When you eat refined carbs and processed foods your metabolism will wreck and you will gain weight and feel sluggish. (Lipman)

CHAPTER 2
WHY AND HOW TO OVERCOME FOOD CRAVINGS

Who has not craved chocolate and eat it like there was no tomorrow? Who has not craved pizza and order it at midnight? In other words, who has not had FOOD CRAVINGS? I used to eat a whole big bag of marshmallows until I was dizzy. Food cravings have little to do with true hunger. Cravings have both biological and psychological components.

The most common cravings are chocolate, salt, sweets, carbohydrates and cheese. We have to understand the causes of food craving to be able to avoid them:

1. Being Dehydrated
Thirst and dehydration make you feel hungry and trigger your cravings.

---

2. Emotional Triggers

Not being happy with your significant other, friends or family, sadness, boredom, stress, poor self esteem, lacking a spiritual life, working out excessively, having a negative body image.

3. Hormonal Changes

Hormonal changes such as during pregnancy, menopause and before your period.

4. When the Gut is Not in Good Shape

When the gut is not in good shape it does not absorb the proper nutrients it needs to produce serotonin, which is the "feel good" neurotransmitter, which has a strong influence on mood, appetite and digestion. Hence the cravings for sugar and carbohydrates such as potato chips or cookies, which increase the release of serotonin, making us feel good temporarily (RJ. Wurtman)

5. Lack of Endorphins

Lack of endorphins, which make us feel good. Endorphins are human-produced opiates that make us feel relaxed. They are produced during sleep and exercise. Eating carbs, sugar and maybe salt increases the production of endorphin in the body. (Morris, et al)

So what do we have to do to avoid craving?

1. Stay Hydrated

Drink water throughout the day to help you stay hydrated and control your hunger. The best way is to have at least two glasses of water when you wake up, during the day and before your meals. Make sure you drink at least half your body weight in pounds in ounces of water; i.e., if you are 150 pounds drink 75 oz of water a day.

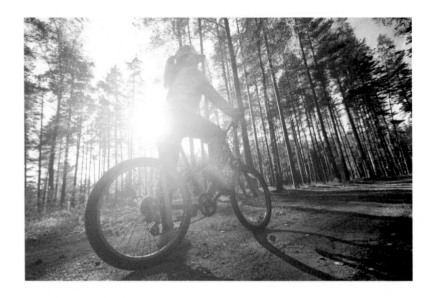

2. Exercise and Sleep

Walk, swim, run, bike whatever you like doing to increase the production of endorphins but make sure you rest too.

3. Eat Something Else

Even if you feel the urge that you need a big chocolate bar, chances are you will feel satisfied with a healthier alternative. That is why I always advice my clients not to have junk food in their houses because they will have a bigger temptation than if they have healthier alternatives.

4. Fresh Vegetable Juices

I also advice my clients to incorporate vegetable juices to avoid sugar cravings. Fresh Vegetable juices – green juices – preferable organic, that you can prepare with a juicer or buy as cold pressed juices which are not processed. They are loaded with natural living enzymes, vitamins, minerals and phytonutrients that will nourish, and heal your body. You do not need to start making major changes in your diet. Just start by adding a green juice everyday and overtime you will find that you do no longer crave those bad foods.

5. Meditation

Take a few minutes every day to meditate, or do something you enjoy.

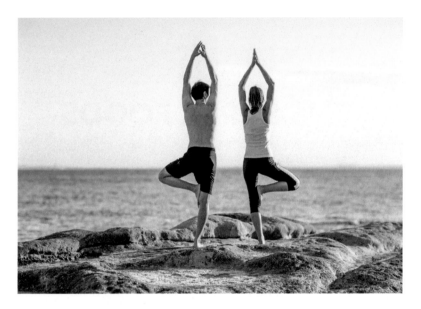

6. Sunshine

10 to 15 Minutes a day of sunshine may boost your serotonin levels so you do not have to reach for comfort foods.

CHAPTER 3

THE SUPER FOODS

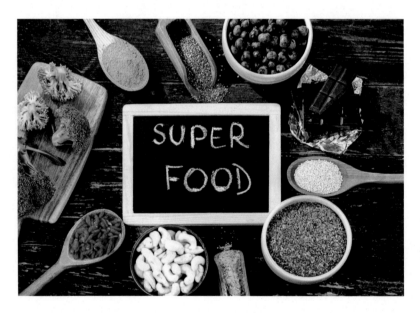

If you are looking for a "magic pill" to look good, boost immunity, feel great and weight loss you can find it in the super foods. Superfood, according to the Oxford Dictionary, is a "nutrient-rich food considered to be specially beneficial for health and well-being."

Hormonal imbalances and inflammation are common conditions in the U.S They are often the culprit behind symptoms such as joint pain, fatigue, high blood pressure, headaches and bloating. Unfortunately, they can also increase the risk of more serious diseases such as cancer and diabetes. The good news is that eating certain foods will help balance your hormones and reduce inflammation. (Syuki)

Here are some of the Super foods and their benefits:

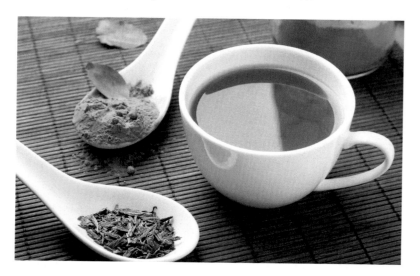

1. Matcha Green Tea

Matcha Green Tea is considered one of the most powerful super foods in the market today. Matcha is the highest quality powdered green tea available. It is high in antioxidants which are the magical nutrients and enzymes responsible for fighting against the negative effects of UV radiation, giving us younger-looking skin, and preventing a number of life threatening maladies. The amazing benefits of Matcha Green Tea are that one bowl provides over 5 times as many antioxidants as any other food. It is loaded with Cathechin. EGC is widely recognized for its anti-cancer fighting properties. Matcha green also enhances calmness.

For over a millennium, Chinese Daoist and Japanese Zen Buddhist monks have used it as a means to relax and meditate while remaining alert. This is due to the amino acid L-Theanine contained in the leaves used to make Matcha. Another side effect of L-Theanine is the production of dopamine and serotonin. These two chemicals serve to enhance mood, improve memory and promote better concentration. Something that we all need but specially of great help when after 40 we begin common menopausal symptoms such as mood changes and problems with memory and concentration. Matcha increases energy levels and endurance, it has also been shown that Matcha increases metabolism and helps the body burn fat about four times faster than average.

Matcha detoxifies the body, capable of naturally removing heavy metals and chemical toxins from the body. The miracle tea also fortifies the immune system. The Catechins in Matcha Green Tea have been shown to have antibiotic properties, which promote overall health. Just one bowl provides substantial quantities of Potassium, Vitamin A and C, Iron, Protein and Calcium. Studies have also shown that people who drink Matcha Green tea on a regular basis have lower cholesterol level of LDL (bad) cholesterol while at the same time they display higher levels of HDL (good) cholesterol. ("10 amazing benefits of Matcha Green Tea")

2. Organic Apples

Organic apples are a natural appetite suppressant. They make you feel satisfied and prevent you from overeating. Packed with fiber and essential vitamins and minerals, they help fight high blood pressure, reduces risk of cancer, fight viral infections and much more. That is why they say, "an apple a day keeps the doctor away." What better snack than half an apple with a tablespoon of almond butter or baked apples for dessert?

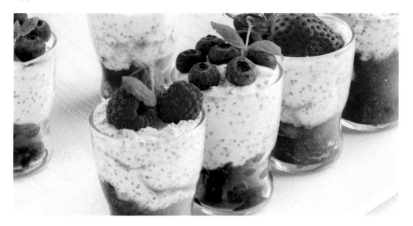

3. Chia Seeds

Chia seeds are the single richest source of plant based omega-3 fatty acids you can buy. They are also loaded with antioxidants, protein and minerals, plus soluble and insoluble fiber to help keep your digestion moving.

Chia seeds also make you feel satisfied helping you to eat less. They are a great alternative for a healthy breakfast or snack. I usually soaked them overnight in almond milk mixed with oatmeal. I add some Goji Berries and top it with fruit such as with bananas, mango puree or a fruit jelly.

4. Maca

Maca benefits both men and women, but I am going to focus on the benefits for women. The most important one is that it decreases menopause symptoms. It has been used extensively as a hormone balancer. Research shows that its high nutrient density and phytochemical content may be the underlying contributor to this effect. Research has shown also that women taking maca enjoyed a reduction in many of the most common menopause symptoms such as hot flashes; sleep disruption, night sweats and depression. It helps to increase the libido because it is loaded with minerals like zinc, iodine and essential fatty acids. Maca may balance sex hormones and may also improve mood. With a good mood and balanced hormones, arousal is usually much easier to achieve.

As women age, it is harder to maintain bone density. Studies of maca's effect on menopausal symptoms have found that it increases important markers associated with bone density. Maca is also rich in vitamins, minerals and fatty acids and proteins. These nutrients naturally support energy levels and aid in recovery from injuries. Studies have shown Maca as safe yet potent super food, which has been a staple in the diet of indigenous people for thousands of years. ("The Truth About Maca.") (Group, "7 Benefits of Maca Root for Women.")

I try having a tablespoon of Maca daily in my oatmeal, protein bar or smoothie.

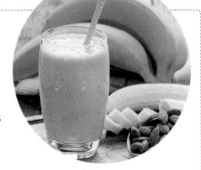

SMOOTHIE

1 cup of almond milk
1 tablespoon of maca
1 tablespoon of goji berries
1 frozen banana

Mix it in the blender or Vitamix and you have a delicious and healthy smoothie.

OATMEAL

1 cup of oatmeal

1 tablespoon of maca

1 tablespoon of Hemp protein

Goji berries

Sliced bananas or any fruit on top

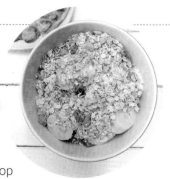

I cook for a few minutes 1 cup of oatmeal in 1 ½ cup of water. When done, I add the maca, goji berries, and the hemp protein. Then to sweeten it, I mix everything with a little teaspoon of Stevia. I top it with sliced bananas, or any kind of fruit. This makes two servings.

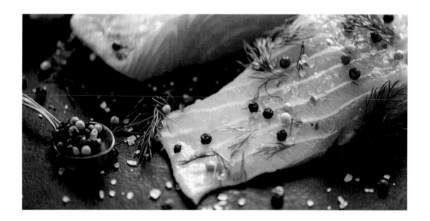

5. Wild Caught Salmon

Wild caught salmon is rich in Omega 3 fatty acids and protein. Intake of fish rich in Omega-3 fat is associated with decreased risk of numerous cardiovascular problems, such as heart attack, stroke, heart arrhythmia, high blood pressure, and high triglycerides in the blood.

It also helps prevent dry eye syndrome, which is a common symptom after 50 and also helps improve your mood and cognition, which really helps during menopause.

Another nutrient found in Wild caught salmon is Selenium, which has been associated with decreased risk of joint inflammation and also with prevention of certain types of cancer. (Zivkovic, et al)

Just make sure you eat wild caught salmon not farmed.

6. Organic Berries

Organic berries such as blueberries contain high antioxidants activity that improve heart health, prevent urinary tract infections, and improve vision.

7. Nuts and Seeds

Nuts and seeds contain high levels of minerals and healthy fats. Walnuts protect your brain and help slow the onset of Alzheimer's and Parkinson's disease. I always advise my clients to eat 10 almonds as a snack, or 30 pistachios. Portion control is key.

8. Leafy Greens

Leafy greens such as spinach, Swiss chard and kale are loaded with fiber, vitamins, minerals and phytochemicals. Every cell you have in your body is benefited from eating leafy greens and the best advantage is that you can eat as much as you want. Spinach boost metabolism and lower insulin levels. (Spritzler)

9. Hemp Protein

Hemp protein is a high fiber protein supplement that can be use to enhance total protein intake for vegans and non-vegans alike. It can be considered a superior protein source due to is above-average digestibility, which also makes it ideal for athletes. Hemp protein additional benefits: potential immune enhancing and anti-fatigue properties, as well as kidney-protective effects.

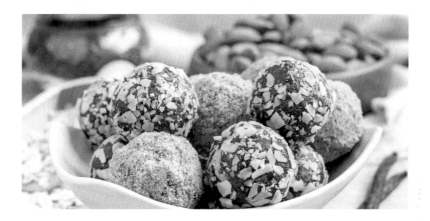

10. Chocolate

At least 70% Dairy free cocoa, or Raw Cacao in moderation, is a delicious treat that actually does your body good. It can help elevate mood, improve blood flow and even lower blood pressure. It helps reduce inflammation and LDL "bad Cholesterol," it is loaded with antioxidants and is delicious!!!

11. Cruciferous Vegetables

If you want to lower your risk of cancer, add broccoli, cauliflower, Brussels sprouts, cabbage, kale and bok choy to your diet. Cruciferous veggies have the ability to inhibit the growth of some types of cancer cells and even stop others by reducing the production of free radicals.

12. Spirulina

Spirulina is made from pond algae. Its top two ingredients are protein and omega fatty acids. I recommend it for people who are vegetarian. Use 1 to 2 teaspoons of spirulina in your daily smoothie or mix with water.

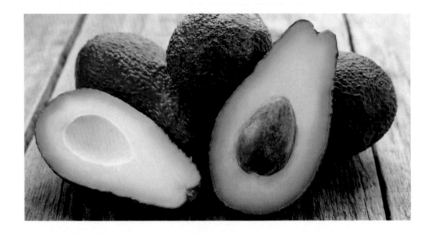

13. Avocado

Avocado has myriads of healthy fats and nutrients such as oleic acid, lutein, folate, vitamin E, monounsaturated fats and glutathione. It can help protect your body from heart disease, cancer, degenerative eye and brain diseases. You can use avocados as a filling for a sandwich with other veggies instead of using cold cuts.

14. Flax Seeds

The lignans (plant compound known as polyphenols) in the flax have been shown to have benefits for menopausal women. It can be used as an alternative to hormone replacement therapy because lignans do have estrogenic properties. These properties may also help reduce the risk of osteoporosis. It can even help menstruating women by helping maintain cycle regularity. The fiber in Flax seeds is effective with eliminating toxins from your body. Also, it makes your hair, skin and nails healthier. Flaxseed is also very helpful to reduce dry eye syndrome, which is very common during and after menopause. Also, a study published in the *Journal of Clinical Cancer* research discovered that consuming Flax seed might decrease the risk of breast cancer. The three lignans found in flaxseeds can be converted into enterolactone and enterodiol by intestinal bacteria, which naturally balance hormones, which may be the reason flax seeds reduce the risk of breast cancer. Another study published in the *Journal of Nutrition* found that lignans in flaxseed might also reduce the risk of endometrial and ovarian cancer. (Pierce, et al)

Consider adding 1 tbsp of flax seed, with a tablespoon of flax seed oil to your smoothie, or 1 tablespoons of flaxseed to your cereal or yoghurt.

It is better to buy the flaxseed and grind it. To keep it fresh save it in an airtight container in the refrigerator. Always drink water with it.

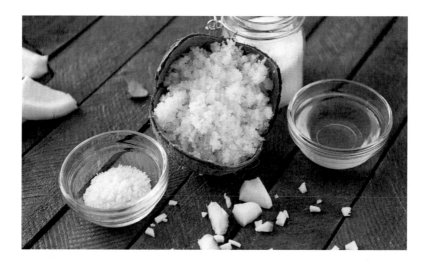

15. Coconut Oil

The fatty acids in this super food fight body fat by converting it into energy that boosts metabolism as opposed to animal derived saturated fats that add body fat. (More on Coconut oil and all of its uses under: "Beauty and Health Tips after 50")

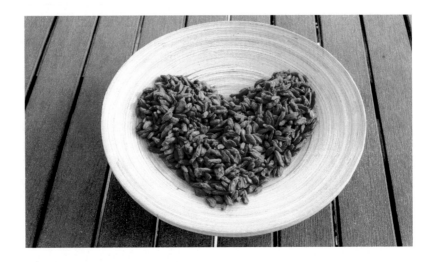

16. Goji Berries

These berries which are delicious are loaded with antioxidants and amino acids, but the real strength lies within their more that 20 vitamins and minerals. These amazing berries have been used for centuries in Asian cultures to strengthen eyesight, fight against viruses, balance hormones, and even to assist with longevity and a healthy life. I add them to acai bowls, to smoothies, to oatmeal, to chia seeds with almond milk and to my Luzkys Protein bars.

17. Beets

Beets are great for men and women after 50, because besides boosting the immune system, they are also considered aphrodisiac. They can increase the blood flow due to their nitrates. Increased blood flow to the genital area is one of the mechanisms Viagra and other pharmaceuticals use to create their effect. Beets also contain high amounts of boron, which is directly related to the production of human sex hormones.

18. Acai

Acai are Brazilian berries usually sold in powder form that are delicious to mix in the blender with frozen bananas as an acai bowl or smoothie. They are loaded with antioxidants that boost your body's energy and ability to focus. Their protein and fiber will also keep you feeling satisfied making the acai berry or powder a weight fighting superhero.

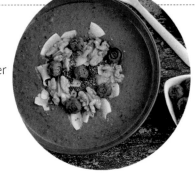

ACAI SMOOTHIE

1 tablespoon of acai powder

1 frozen banana

Organic blueberries (I use organic frozen)

½ a cup of almond milk

½ cup of water

1 tablespoon of maca

Mix everything together in the Vitamix or blender.

19. Oatmeal

One of my favorite carbs is oatmeal. I love it because beside being delicious is low in calories; a cup has approximately 130 calories.

It also stays in your stomach longer, making you feel satisfied. Oatmeal will make you feel less hunger and have fewer cravings. It provides high levels of fiber, low levels of fat and high levels of protein. It stabilizes blood sugar and reduces risk of diabetes (type2). The high fiber and complex carbohydrates slow down the conversion of this whole food to simple sugars. The high levels of magnesium nourish the body's proper use of glucose and insulin secretion. Oatmeal removes your bad cholesterol without affecting you good cholesterol. Many studies have shown that the unique fiber content in oatmeal, called beta-glucan, has beneficial effects on cholesterol levels. Another benefit of oatmeal is that is contains lignans, which protect against heart disease and cancer. One lignan, called enterolactone, is though to protect against breast and other hormone-dependent cancers as well as heart disease. A study at Tuft University shows that the unique antioxidants in oatmeal called avenanthramides, help prevent free radicals from damaging LDL cholesterol, thus reducing the risk of cardiovascular disease. It also enhances immune response to disease.

When you buy oatmeal make sure you buy regular oatmeal not the instant oatmeal, which is processed. The regular oatmeal retains its nutrients and is slower to digest. It will also be slower to cook.

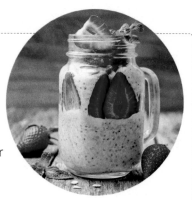

OVERNIGHT OATMEAL AND CHIA SEEDS

Half a cup of oatmeal
1 tablespoon of chia seeds
Almond milk, coconut milk or
cashew milk
Goji berries

Soak the oatmeal, the chia seeds and the goji berries overnight in the nut milk. The next day you can eat them with any kind of fruit on top such as bananas, organic strawberries or mango.

POST WORKOUT MEAL

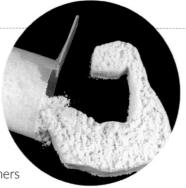

Half a cup of cooked
oatmeal in water
1 serving of whey protein
isolate with no antibiotics or
BGH and no artificial sweeteners
Goji berries
1 tablespoon of maca
8 ounces of water

Mix everything together in the Vitamix or blender.

CHAPTER 4
SYMPTOMS OF MENOPAUSE

Most women will experience some symptoms around menopause. The duration and severity of these symptoms varies from woman to woman.

Symptoms usually start a few months or years before your periods stop, known as the perimenopause, and can persist some time afterwards. On average, most symptoms last around four years from your last period. However, 1 in every 10 women experiences them for 12 years.

If you experience the menopause suddenly rather than gradually for example, as a result of cancer treatment, your symptoms may worsen.

A change in the normal pattern of your period is one of the signs of menopause. You may start having heavy periods or unusually light.

Also the frequency of the periods may also be affected. Eventually you will stop having periods all together. ("Menopause - Symptoms")

("Menopause - Symptoms and Types of Menopause")

Common menopausal symptoms:

- Hot flashes- short sudden feelings of heat, usually in the face neck and chest, which can make your skin red and sweaty.

- Difficulty sleeping, which may make you feel tired and irritable during the day. If you add a workout routine every day and avoid taking naps during the day this could easily be fix.

- A reduced sex drive (libido). That is why I recommend adding to your diet all the super foods, such as beets and maca. In addition, I think it has to do with the way you feel because of all the hormonal changes going on in your body. That is why it is so important to stop eating processed foods, meats and dairy that contain hormones, which add more load to your body. Also having an active lifestyle helps because working out produces endorphins in your body that make you feel good and if you feel good overall you will also feel good sexually.

- Problems with memory and concentration.

- Vaginal dryness and pain, itching and discomfort during sex- (add some coconut oil to your foreplay).

- Headaches.

- Mood swings, such as low mood or anxiety.

- Palpitations.

- Joint stiffness, aches and pains, which also happen to men.

- Reduced muscles mass and therefore slower metabolism.

- Recurrent urinary infections such as cystitis.

- It can also increase your risk of developing osteoporosis, therefore the importance of proper nutrition.

Through loving myself, eating clean, loving sports, being blessed by having wonderful parents, amazing sons that have given me so much happiness, real friends, and a spiritual life, I have been able not to feel any of these symptoms. After my own experience and dealing with clients who show great results after following my advice, I decided to write this book to be able to share my knowledge and experience. I want to create a "ripple effect" like Joshua Rosenthal, the founder of IIN, taught me. I want everybody to learn how to prevent disease and LOOK AND FEEL FABULOUS AFTER 50!

CHAPTER 5
LOOK AND FEEL FABULOUS!

SO, WHAT DO WE HAVE TO DO TO LOOK AND FEEL FABULOUS AFTER 50?

Just as with any big change, it can take some time to get used to. It is the long-term accumulation of small decisions and daily actions that will make you see a change to leading a healthy and active life. It is not about a fad diet that will make you lose weight and rejuvenate you 10 years; it is not about going to a spa for one week that will forever change your life, or a liposuction that will give you a flat stomach. It is not only one thing that will make you feel revitalized, younger or better. It is about adopting habits and patterns of living that are associated with a healthy, happy and vigorous active life. That means, for example, that adding just a fitness class such as Spinning or Zumba is not enough. It is about changing your lifestyle. It is about having good and positive relationships, loving yourself, doing things you enjoy, being active, learning new things, eating healthy, enjoying life, and last but not least, being thankful for everything you have. Personally, I start my day by giving thanks for three things that are good in my life and by repeating my mantra "Day by day, I am doing better and better in every way." (Émile Coué) It is not what you sometimes do; it is who you are.

So How Do I Start?

1. Start by Drinking More Water

Our body is about 60% water. We are constantly losing water via urine and sweat. The health authorities recommend 8-ounce glasses per day. (Popkin, et al)("Hydration FAQs") However, there are other health "gurus" like me who think we are always on the brink of dehydration and we need to sip water constantly throughout the day, even when we are not thirsty.

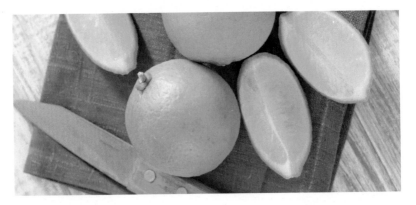

Water needs also depends on the individual activities and the weather. I recommend starting your day by drinking 1 glass of water and another glass of warm water with lemon or lime juice. Warm lemon or lime water in the morning cleanses and detoxifies your body. Lemon is known to have strong antiviral, antibacterial and immune-boosting properties. It is loaded with Vitamin C, which will help your system internally and will also reflect in the beautification of your skin.

When putting this into practice, make sure that it is purified water to avoid additives like fluoride. Also, make sure that it is luke warm water rather than boiling hot. It is a digestive aid because lemon flushes out unwanted materials and toxins from the body. Lemon have a de-bloating property, which can help relieve indigestion issues like heartburn, belching and bloating.

The American Cancer Society recommends warm lemon water to cancer sufferers to help stimulate bowel movements. Lemons also increase the rate of urination in the body. Therefore, toxins are released at a faster rate and you can also enjoy a healthier urinary tract health. Drinking warm lemon or lime water in the morning also is a great pH balancer. Even though lemons are acidic, they are one of the most alkalizing foods for the body. Diseases only occur when the body pH is acidic. Drinking lemon or lime water regularly can help to remove overall acidity in the body, including uric acid in the joints, which is one of the primary causes of pain and inflammation. Another perk for drinking lemon or limewater is fresh breath.

However, the only downfall of drinking lemon water is that citric acid erodes tooth enamel, so to avoid this, brush your teeth before you drink your lemon or lime water to leave a protective coat on your teeth, and if you are in a hurry, you can swish with pure water after you are done with your lemon or lime water drink.

This miracle drink is also an energy and mood enhancer. The energy a human receives from foods comes from the atoms and molecules in the food. A reaction occurs when the positive charged ions from food enter the digestive tract and interacts with the negative charged enzymes. Lemon and limes are one of the few foods that contain more negative charged ions, providing your body with more energy when it enters the digestive tract. And last but not least, drinking warm lemon or lime water as soon as you wake up is a weight loss aid. It helps you feel fuller longer, thanks to their high pectin fiber content, which helps fight hunger cravings. Studies have shown that people who maintain a more alkaline diet do lose weight faster. (Grussi)

If you are trying to lose weight, I advise you to drink 8-16 ounces of water before your meals. This will make you consume fewer calories, which can ultimately lead to weight loss. The water provides a sense of fullness, so not as much food is needed to reach the point of satiety.

Benefits of drinking water: increases energy and avoid fatigue, promotes weight loss, flushes out toxins, improves skin complexion, maintains regularity, boost immune system, prevents cramps and sprains, and finally, it is a natural headache remedy.

2. Avoid Processed Foods

Processed foods that claim they are low fat, low carbs, vitamin fortified, no trans fat, contain Vitamin C, etc are an illusion, often appearing to be healthy. These foods that are loaded with chemicals and preservatives are the cause of coronary heart disease, obesity, diabetes, stroke and cancer. ("Top 10 Cancer Causing Foods")

The food industry adds lots of salt, sugar and oil to make it taste good. When you eat white bread and other foods that are made with white flour, which is highly processed, you are basically consuming empty calories with no nutrition at all. I teach my clients that rather than counting calories, watching fat grams or reducing carbs for "healthy eating" simply eat whole foods. As Michael Polan states, they are more the product of nature than the "product of industry."

Making smarter food choices by avoiding processed foods will reduce health care costs later in life, and it will make you experience great health benefits such as having more energy, lose weight, and feel healthier overall. When you start eating real foods your taste buds will not like to go back to processed foods.

1. Do not eat anything that contains more than 5 ingredients or ingredients you can not pronounce.

2. Do not eat anything that contains preservatives and can be on the shelves of supermarkets forever.

3. Always Read Labels

The best advice one can give as a nutritionist, is to always read the ingredient list. All packaged foods come with a nutrition label meant to provide you with the information necessary to know what you are eating. Understanding what is in the food you eat helps you make healthier food choices. It is the only way to truly know what is in your food and how processed it is. It takes time, but if you want to stop eating the wrong foods, you have to do it.

Do not let the words "fat free," healthy," "refined," "fortified" or "enriched" mislead you into buying processed foods that are not nutritious. We do not know how these chemicals additions given to processed foods, will affect our metabolism in the long run.

From my experience, with dealing with clients who want to lose weight, when they stop eating processed foods and drink more water right away, they start losing weight because their metabolism start working as it should.

4. Breaking the Rules

Stick to the rule of good eating 90% of the time and splurge 10% of the time. I love the word splurge because when you splurge you are treating yourself to something you really want. Whether is a day at the spa, an expensive bag or a hot chocolate lava cake; everyone needs to splurge in life and enjoy it while you are doing it. JUST MAKE SURE YOUR SPLURGE makes up less than 10 % of your meals each week.

5. Shopping

Avoid temptations to eat a bag of fried chips or candy by keeping junk food out of the house. My children always used to ask me "Mommy, when are you going to buy some junk food?" This is important to keep in mind specially if you are the one doing the grocery shopping.

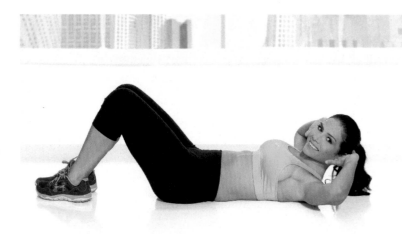

6. Exercise

Do you want to boost your metabolism, feel better, have more energy and perhaps even live longer? Exercise.

According to Mayo Clinic, the health benefits of regular exercise and physical activity are:

- **Exercise controls weight.** Exercise can help prevent excess weight gain. When you engage in physical activity you burn calories. The more intense the activity the more calories you burn but this does not mean you are allowed to eat junk food. If you can not find the time for an actual workout, get more active through the day in simple ways by taking the stairs instead of the elevator, walking or biking instead of driving.

- **Exercise combats health conditions and diseases** such as depression, certain types of cancer, arthritis, diabetes, heart disease, and high blood pressure.

- **Exercise improves mood.** Physical activity stimulates various brain chemicals that may leave you feeling happier and more relaxed. You may also feel better about your appearance and yourself when you exercise regularly which improves your self esteem.

- **Exercise boost energy.** Regular physical activity can improve your muscle strength and boost your endurance. Exercise and physical activity deliver oxygen and nutrients to your tissues and help your cardiovascular system work more efficiently.

- **Exercise promotes better sleep.**

- **Exercise puts the spark back into your sex life.** Regular physical activity can leave you feeling energized and looking better, which may have a positive effect in your sex life. Regular physical activity can lead to enhanced arousal for women, and men who exercise are less likely to have problems with erectile dysfunction than are men who do not exercise.

- **Exercise is fun.** Most of my best friends are my tennis and bicycle buddies. Working out or doing a sport we like and enjoy is an excellent way to connect with family and friends in a fun social setting. Find a physical activity you enjoy and just do it.

Exercise and physical activity are a great way to feel better and have fun while enjoying the benefits of gaining health. As a general goal, aim to do at least 30 minutes of physical activity per day, but if you want to lose weight or meet specific fitness goals, you may need to exercise more. Remember to always check with your doctor before beginning any exercise program, specially, if you have not exercise for a long time, have a chronic health problem or have any concerns.

7. Love Yourself.

Dedicate time to do things you enjoy and always keep learning. After 50 most of us have already raised a family. Children are gone and we have more time to dedicate to ourselves. So, why not learn something new? Try a new sport? Travel to places you have never been? Donate your time to help others who are not as fortunate as we are?

The most valuable commodity in life is TIME. We ask ourselves how did time went by so fast? I never thought I would be 50, Where did time go? I just blinked my eyes and time went by tooooo fast. I used to see the beauty queen contestant as old women; doctors were old; now I see them like young people. Everything is relative. One of the teachings of Buddhism is that nothing is forever - Impermanence. Do not leave what you want to do or experiment for tomorrow.
Start today.

CHAPTER 6
HOW TO BOOST YOUR METABOLISM AFTER 50

Your metabolism includes all the things your body does to turn food into energy and keep you going. Some people have a faster metabolism than others. Some things that affect your metabolism include things you can not control such as aging, sex and genes. According to the article "How to Boost your metabolism with exercise", we have to focus on what really makes a difference: Exercise. Exercise becomes even more important as you get older. As we age we naturally lose muscle mass, which slows down our metabolism. Working out can stop that slide. It is simple. You need to challenge your muscles in two ways:

1. Amp Your Workout
Any kind of exercise, whether you are riding your bike or running, burns calories. Make it more intense and you will burn more calories. Try doing interval training such as switching back and forth between higher and lower intensity such as walking for 3 minutes and then

running one minute, or biking in a low gear with a higher cadence and then switching to a high gear making it more intense. You make it really challenging and then back down to your own pace, and repeat. Also, when lifting weights, I recommend switching from doing 3 sets of 12-15 reps each; for example, leg press exercises to 3 minutes running in the treadmill, then go to 3 sets of 12-15 reps of leg extensions to 3 minutes in the bike and so on. Another kind of workout routine that help you lose fat is weight training and then finishing up with 20 to 40 minutes of cardio. If you are new to working out, I would recommend you to hire a Personal Trainer who will help you find out what will be the best routine according to your own personal needs. The important thing is to find an activity you enjoy doing. Also, I recommend cross training which means combining exercises to work various parts of the body or doing different kinds of sports such as running, bicycling, swimming, taking a fitness class or strength training. Alternative forms of exercise have definite benefits: improves fitness, builds strength, and avoids boredom from doing the same activity.

2. Build Muscle

Your body constantly burns calories, even when you are doing nothing. This resting metabolic rate is much higher in people with more muscle. Every pound of muscle uses about 6 calories a day, while each pound of fat burns only 2 calories daily. That small difference can add over time. After a strength training session muscles are activated all over your body, raising your average daily metabolic rate. In terms of fat loss, strength training is the best way to increase your lean muscle mass and burn more calories. Most forms of resistance exercise will increase your calorie expenditure, even in the hours post exercise.

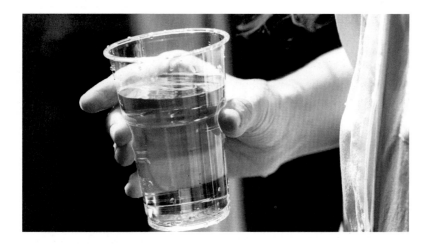

3. Drink Water

Your body needs water to process calories. If you are even mildly dehydrated, your metabolism may slow down. Stay hydrated and drink at least eight glasses of water per day, preferably before each meal or snack and when you wake up.

4. Protein

Your body burns more calories digesting protein than it does eating fat or carbohydrates. Good sources of protein include lean organic beef, wild caught fish, organic chicken, nuts, beans, organic eggs and yoghurt.

5. Eating More Often Can Help You Lose Weight

When you eat large meals with many hours in between, your metabolism slows down between meals. Having a small meal every 3 to 4 hours keeps your metabolism cranking, so you burn more calories over the course of the day. Several studies have also shown that people who snack regularly eat less at mealtime.

6. Eat Spicy Foods

Another way of boosting your metabolism is by eating spicy foods that have natural chemicals that can kick your metabolism into higher gear. Use cayenne pepper, red or green chili peppers as spices to boost your metabolic rate.

RECIPE FOR BOOSTING YOUR METABOLISM

1 tablespoon of organic apple vinegar

A pinch or cayenne pepper

1 squeezed lime or lemon

Mix in a glass of warm water.

Drink when you wake up in the morning.

---

7. Coffee

I love coffee because of the energy and concentration perks I get from it. Caffeine taken in moderation can help you feel less tired and even increase your endurance while you exercise. Besides these benefits, it also gives you a short-term rise in your metabolic rate.

8. Green Tea

Adding green tea to your diet offers the combined benefits of caffeine and catechins, substances shown to rev up the metabolism. Research suggest that drinking 2 to 4 cups of green tea may push the body to burn 17 % more calories during moderately intense exercise for a short time. ("Green Tea Boosts Metabolism, Protects Against Diseases")

9. Do Not Do Crash Diets

Avoid diets involving eating fewer than 1200 calories (if you are a woman) or 1800 calories per day (if you are a man). These kinds of diets make you lose muscle, which in turns slows your metabolism. The final result is that your body burns fewer calories and gains weight faster than before the diet. ("How to Boost your metabolism with exercise")

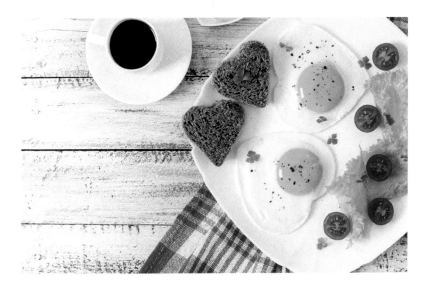

10. Breakfast

Always, always have breakfast. It is the most important meal of the day. It kick-starts your metabolism, helping you burn calories during the day. It also gives you the energy you need to get things done and helps you focus at work or at school. Skipping the morning meal can throw off you body's rhythm of fasting and eating, When you wake up, the blood sugar your body needs to make your muscles and brain work their best is usually low. Breakfast helps replenish it. If your body does not get that fuel from food, you may feel zapped of energy and you will be more likely to overeat later in the day. So, do not give me the excuse that you are not hungry when you wake up, or that you only had a cup of coffee. Most of the people who do not eat breakfast that come to me usually have weight problems and lack of energy. It is better to eat a small piece of fruit or some yogurt and then later eat something more substantial, especially if you workout early in the morning.

More tips!

1. Eating Out

Many people tell me it is hard to eat healthy because they travel often and eat at restaurants a lot. Here is my advice on eating out tips: when you go to a restaurant avoid the breadbasket and the butter, unless you really want to splurge because the bread that was served is unique or is whole grain bread. Just brainwash your way of thinking by asking yourself why should I eat white processed bread that is only full of empty calories that will give me a fat belly? To avoid the temptation just ask the waiter not to bring the breadbasket. Also, if you are trying to lose weight please abstain from eating carbs after 6 pm. When you order from the menu, avoid creamy sauces on top of the main plate. If they come with sauces, order it on the side. Do the same with the salad dressing. Order it on the side, and just use a little. It is preferably to order the salad dressing that is made with olive or avocado oil and vinegar instead of a rich creamy sauce made with mayonnaise. Ask if the fish they are serving is wild caught, and if they do not have wild caught do not order it. This will be good for your health and will also make restaurant owners avoid serving farmed fish, which is detrimental to our health and to the environment. You can order grilled organic meats to avoid sauces and deep fried foods. Last and not least, avoid the dessert unless is your splurge day (the 10% rule) or just do like the French do, have a little portion and share (Portion Control.)

2. Eating In a Plane

Usually, food that is served on airplanes is not good, unless you are traveling in one of the top ten airlines of the world where you can choose the meal according to your needs. I usually travel with nuts and fruits in case I do not like what they serve.

3. Eat Slowly - Chew Your Food

According to the article "Take a light stroll", digestion initially begins in the mouth. As you start to chew your food, digestive enzymes found in saliva begin to break it down, preparing for nutrient absorption. It's important to chew your food thoroughly to achieve maximum absorption of all your vitamins and minerals.

How to Chew Properly

To get into the habit of chewing foods thoroughly:

1. Try counting the chews in each bite, aiming for 30 to 50 times, until the food becomes liquid.

2. Try putting your utensils down between bites to help you better concentrate on chewing.

3. When you eat, do not do other things, such as reading or watching television. Just enjoy your food.

Chewing breaks down food and makes it easier on the stomach and small intestine.

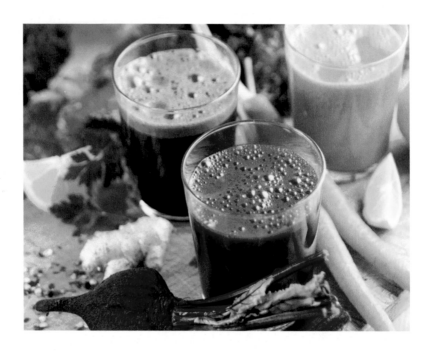

4. Juicing

Fresh vegetable juices like green juice are loaded with natural living enzymes, vitamins, minerals and phytonutrients that will nourish and heal your body. Fresh vegetable and green juices are low in sugar, alkalizing, cleansing/detoxifying and restorative. These fresh juices activate/repair dormant and diseased cells: allowing your body to fight diseases, such as cancer. As proof, Kris Carr, New York Times best selling author was able to completely heal herself from a rare and incurable stage 4 of cancer. She did this all by eating a plant based and daily green juices. There are many studies that show how people were able to reverse many incurable diseases and illness by going plant based and drinking fresh green juice. (Stein)(Mcdougall)

The other advantage of adding green juices to your diet, is that it prevents you from having sugar cravings and also helps you stop eating processed foods.

You do not need to make major changes to your diet, just start by incorporating a fresh green juice every day.

A great way to start your day is by having a green juice in the morning. Leafy greens contain chlorophyll. The molecular structure of chlorophyll is almost identical to the hemoglobin in our blood. While the center atom of hemoglobin is iron, the center atom of chlorophyll is magnesium. This similar composition allows chlorophyll to actually rebuild and replenish our blood cells while delivering oxygen to our tissues. It also acts as a chelator, which pulls toxic heavy metals from our body and has anti-carcinogenic properties, protecting against cancer-causing substances such as cooked meat toxins and air pollution. Starting your day with a green juice will make you feel energized, will help you avoid sugar cravings during the day, and you will get a big boost of alkalizing minerals, oxygen and enzymes.

You will find that over time you will no longer crave bad foods. A green juice a day is all it takes to make a BIG change in your health.

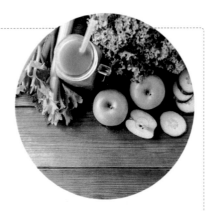

GREEN JUICE

1 peeled lime or lemon
1 organic green apple
1 peeled cucumber
Organic spinach
Organic parsley
Ginger

5. Eat 5 Times a Day

When I tell people to eat 5 times a day sometimes they freak out. They think they are going to gain weight. We are not talking about

5 big meals we are talking about 3 meals a day and 2 healthy snacks. If you do this, you will keep your metabolism going strong and your energy levels will remain constant. It will reduce your food cravings and feel less hunger. If you just have an early breakfast at 7am and then a big lunch at 1pm, you are going to be starving; you will eat anything, eat too much, your blood sugar will drop and you will feel tired. Because you feel tired after eating a lot, you will crave sugar to feel better and it becomes a vicious cycle. To prevent this, I recommend to my clients depending on their needs to eat breakfast, a midmorning healthy snack, lunch, a mid-afternoon healthy snack and dinner.

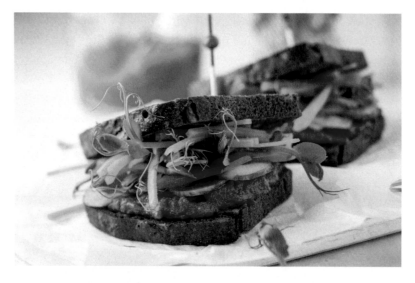

6. Eat More Raw Foods

Raw Foods are whole foods that have not been refined chemically, processed, denatured or heated above 118° F (48°C), so its nutritional content is preserved. The major raw foods are fruits, vegetables, sprouted seed, nuts, grains, sea vegetables and natural fats. Fundamentally, raw foods are not a new concept. Various government and health organizations tell us we need to eat several servings of fruits and vegetables per day. When we eat foods in their natural and uncooked state, we receive all the vitamins, minerals, phytonutrients and enzymes Mother Nature intended for us. When foods are cooked almost 70 per cent of these nutrients are lost.

The benefits of raw foods are:

- They are energizing. Most people notice their energy levels increasing when they eat raw. Raw foods are easier to digest so less strain is put on the body to produce its own digestive enzymes.

- Raw Foods are hydrating. This can help us with sluggishness, dry skin and false hunger when we do not consume enough water.

- Raw foods help boost our immune system. Raw foods contain copious amounts of Vitamin C, beta-carotene and zinc, which are three very powerful immune boosters.

- Raw foods contain loads of fiber, which is essential for sweeping the digestive tract of waste. Incorporating raw foods in your diet will make you go to the bathroom regularly.

- Raw foods contain phytonutrients such as Lycopene and Resveratrol. These are plant chemical compounds that act as antioxidants, immune boosters and hormone stabilizers, which produces many health benefits such as detoxifying the liver, preventing heart disease and cancer, and protecting our eyes from macular degeneration.

You do not need to be a vegetarian or vegan to go Raw, nor do you need to be 100 percent Raw to reap all the benefits. Any amount of raw food is beneficial, but try to aim for a 50% raw diet to feel a notable difference. If you add just a vegetable juice to your morning routine, incorporate at least two pieces of fruits per day, nuts as snacks and a salad at lunch and dinner, you will feel the difference and the benefits of incorporating raw foods in your diet.

Adopting a plant-based diet is compassionate. Eating less meat means you participate in less animal suffering. The conditions for animals raised in Factory farms are very sad and cruel. They are raised in packed conditions where they can hardly move. Many stand in their own manure and never go out and see the daylight. Chickens have their beaks clipped because they go mad and attack each other. They are fed with unnatural diets. They are given tons of hormones and antibiotics so they do not get sick and survive in the deplorable conditions in which they live. If we can get most of our nutrients from plants and we can avoid many diseases such as cancer, diabetes, high blood pressure, high cholesterol, and heart problems, why not start eating more plant based foods? If you enjoy meat and eggs, buy grass fed meats and pastured eggs from farmers who have made a commitment to raising their animals in a compassionate way. (Wignall)

One of the biggest concerns people have about following a plant-based diet is whether they will get enough protein. All plants contain protein, especially green leafy vegetables such as kale, spinach, parsley, arugula, and collard greens. They are composed of 35 to 50 percent protein. Other good quality sources of protein include hemp seeds, goji berries, cacao, almonds, bee pollen, spirulina, chia seeds, chlorella, blue-green algae, pumpkin seeds, sprouts, sprouted grains, sprouted wild rice, and vegetable powders.

Sources of vegetable protein

Hemp Seeds	1 ounce	10 grams
Almonds	¼ cup	7 grams
Buckwheat	1 cup	6 grams
Chia Seeds	¼ cup	6 grams
Cacao Nibs	1 ounce	4 grams
Goji Berries	1 ounce	4 grams
Kale	1 cup	2.5 grams
Spinach	1 cup	2 grams

7. Avoid Eating Soy Products

Avoid eating soy products such as soymilk, tofu and imitation meats made of soy. Soy contains phytoestrogens and various toxins that can have a profound effect on the thyroid and the hormonal development of children as well as many other health problems in women such as breast cancer. Soy consumption also is harmful for men because it lowers the testosterone levels and increases the estrogen levels causing lower libido, producing obesity and abnormal enlargement of the mammary glands, gynecomastia. In addition, most nonorganic soybeans are genetically modified organism (GMOs) which have unknown health risk. GMOs can cause infertility, allergic reactions, and metabolic disruptions and may be linked to liver failure.

I see an alarming amount of people consuming soy protein drinks that substitute a meal and soymilk every day. Babies being fed with soy formula thinking it is healthy, when in reality is detrimental to our health. The only soy that is good to consume is the fermented organic soy, which does not do harm such as Tempeh, Miso and traditionally soy sauces such as Tamari and Nama Shoyu.

8. Portion Distortion

Are you a member of the clean plate club? Were you brainwashed when you were little to eat everything in your plate because there were kids in India dying of hunger? Although your parents meant good, this was not necessarily good. We should only eat until we are satisfied.

How much we eat is all too often dependent on how much we are served. The more on our plate, the more we eat – bigger portions can cause people to eat 30% to 50% more than they usually would! (Neporent) (Young)(Scott)

We should follow these portion control tips:

- *Use smaller containers.* Separate leftovers into single serving containers so you're less tempted to eat all the remains.

- *Have a salad or vegetable soup before your meal.* It will curb your appetite and give you a sense of satiety.

- *Split an entrée with a friend or with your significant other.* When eating out, ask a friend or your significant other to share a single entrée!

- *Buy or make single serving snacks.* You can easily portion out a large container of almonds into individual bags. You'll be less likely to go back for another baggie than reach in for another handful.

- *Keep seconds out of sight.* Leave the food in the kitchen to avoid refill temptations.

- *Have mini meals throughout the day.* This will keep you satisfied and decrease the urge to eat large portions at traditional mealtimes.

We think that eating is only to promote or maintain bodily health, but according to Michael Polan, there are many other reasons to eat food: "pleasure, social community, identity, and ritual. Health is not the only thing going on our plates."

Families traditionally ate together, around a table and not a TV, and at regular meal times. Nowadays, because of different time schedules, we are not able to share all of our   meals with our family, but at least it would be good to have dinner together. Having meals together is a time to be able to share the day experiences with your loved ones.

CHAPTER 7
BEAUTY AND HEALTH TIPS AFTER 50

A lot of skin care products on the market today contain chemicals that the body finds unable to use or hard to eliminate. They tend to build up in the deeper skin layers, not only interfering with internal cleansing, but also restricting the skin's ability to absorb natural nutrients. (Ertl)

That is why it is so important to use natural products. There are apps that you can download on your phone such as THINK DIRTY (go to the App store in your iPhone and download the Think Dirty App, which is free) where you can search or scan any beauty product such as make up, body lotions, shampoos, etc. It will show you by a dirty meter the carcinogenicity, developmental, reproductive toxicity, allergies and immunotoxicities levels of each product giving a grade from 1 -10 being 10 the dirtiest. It also shows the list of the ingredients it contains, showing which ingredients are toxic to your body and which ones are ok to use. It also shows you a list of alternative products you can use instead. So, for example, if you are buying a hand cream brand x, you search it or scan it in the app. If they give it a grade of 10, you can look for different brands of hand creams with a grade of 0, which are safe to use.

One of the worst ingredients that is widely used for body lotions, make up, shaving creams, deodorants and tanning lotions are parabens. Parabens are man-made preservative chemicals used by manufacturers because they are cost effective. They have serious health side effects such as:

1. Interfering with the functioning of the endocrine system. Parabens are endocrine disruptors stored in the body tissue that interferes with glandular activity and hormone production. Moreover these preservative chemicals are associated with the following in infants and children: developmental disorders, dysfunction of the immune system, learning problem and well as reproductive disorders. (Tacon)

2. Parabens cause premature aging. Ironically, while several of the beauty products are sold to enhance the skin, such as moisturizers and lotions, research has found that they accelerate the skin aging process. As reported by live-naturally.co.uk, researchers for, the Kyoto Prefectural University of Medicine in Japan found that the methyl type of Parabens increase sensitivity and damages the skin when exposed to ultraviolet rays. Skin cells die at a much faster rate than normal.

3. Pseudo-Estrogen Effects: In 2004, a finding from a study published in the "Journal of Applied Toxicology " were released indicating that parabens may play a role in the development of certain types of breast cancer. Specifically, parabens act like estrogen, which may increase the risk of women developing estrogen-positive breast cancer.

One of the reasons I was motivated to write this book was because in my family my mother and two sisters have had estrogen-positive breast tumors.

4. Male Reproductive Effects – In addition to this chemical's estrogen-like effects in women, there has been several studies that link parabens (live-naturally.co.uk) to adversely interfering with the male reproductive system such as low sperm count as well as decreased levels of testosterone in men, and it was concluded that these results were related to the absorption of parabens in commercial products.

Before buying any beauty product, make sure you read the list of ingredients and AVOID purchasing any that contains PARABENS.

1. Body Brushing

You may be thinking, *Why do I need to add something else to my already busy morning routine?* Let me assure you, the extra five minutes this takes is well worth the investment.

The largest organ in the body is the skin. It is one of the most important elimination organs in the body, playing a large role in daily detoxification. The skin receives a third of all the blood that is circulated in the body. When the blood is full of toxic materials, the skin will reflect this problem.

According to Lee Sutherland in his article "Why You Should Start Dry Body Brushing Today", the benefits of dry skin brushing include: Increases the circulation to the skin. This could possibly reduce the appearance of cellulite. Cellulite is toxic material accumulated in your body's fat cells. So, rather than take drastic measures like liposuction, how about utilizing the dry skin brushing

- Dry body brushing helps shed dead skin cells and encourages new cell renewal, which results in smoother and brighter skin. It can also help with any pesky ingrown hairs.

- It assists in improving vascular blood circulation and lymphatic drainage. By releasing toxins, it encourages the body's discharge of metabolic wastes so the body is able to run more effectively.

- Dry skin brushing rejuvenates the nervous system by stimulating nerve endings in the skin (and it feels pretty great, too!).

- It helps with muscle tone and gives you a more even distribution of fat deposits.

- Dry skin brushing helps your skin to absorb nutrients by eliminating clogged pores.

To reap all the benefits of Dry Skin Brushing, all you need to do is purchase a natural bristle brush (not one made from nylon or synthetic materials). One with a long handle is also a plus, as it means you can reach all areas of the body.

The directions are pretty simple:

- Start on dry skin before bathing.

- Work in gentle circular, upward motions, then longer, smoother strokes.

- Always begin at the ankles in upwards movements towards the heart - the lymphatic fluid flows through the body towards the heart, so it's important that you brush in the same direction.

- Your back is the only exception to the preceding rule; brush from the neck down to the lower back.

- After you've finished with the ankles, move up to the lower legs, thighs, stomach, back and arms. Be cautious of softer and sensitive skin around the chest and breasts, and never brush over inflamed skin, sores, sun-burnt skin, or skin cancer.

- Ensure you shower to wash away the dead skin cells and impurities.

- Tip: alternating temperatures in the shower from hot to cold will further invigorate the skin and stimulate blood circulation, bringing more blood to the outer layers of the skin.

- Then, follow it up with a slick moisturizer to nourish the skin (personally, I'm a fan of coconut oil).

- Give it a go for 30 consecutive days and your body will love you for it!

2. Massage

To look and feel better, have a regular massage. Massage is a general term for pressing, rubbing and manipulating your skin, muscles, tendons and ligaments. The benefits of having a massage are: encourages relaxation, improves circulation, improves posture, lowers blood pressure, relaxes muscles, and improves flexibility and range of motion.

3. Facial Treatments

Have a facial treatment regularly. Besides enjoying the pampering and relaxation you feel when receiving a facial treatment, facial treatments have a multitude of other benefits such as deep cleaning your skin, moisturize and relieve stress. Facial treatments help to improve and restore circulation to facial skin layers, increasing the flow of oxygen-enriched blood to skin cells. This rush of blood to the skin gives your skin a healthy glow and plumps skin cells with vital nutrients and water, which reduces the appearances of wrinkles and dry skin. ("What are the Benefits of Facial Treatments")

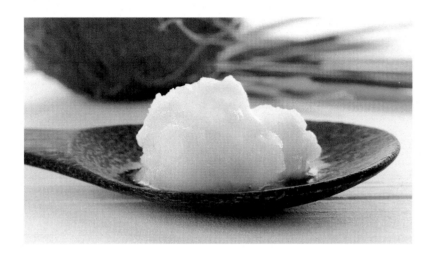

4. Organic Coconut Oil

According to the article "Health Benefits of Coconut oil", Coconut Oil has a multitude of health benefits, which include but are not limited to skin care, hair care, improving digestion and immunity against a host of infections and diseases.

Health Benefits of Coconut oil:

Skin Care

Coconut oil is an excellent moisturizer, which works as a massage oil. It does not have any adverse side effects on the skin. It is used to prevent dryness and flaking of skin. It also delays the appearance of wrinkles and sagging of skin, which normally accompany aging. It also helps in treating skin problems such as dermatitis, psoriasis, eczema and other skin infections. It can also be use to remove make up and be use as a lip moisturizer. As a scrub, I mix it with sugar. It helps me get rid of dead skin cells and leaves the skin soft and lubricated.

Hair Care

Coconut oil helps in healthy growth of hair and gives your hair a shiny quality. The day before I wash my hair I massage it on my hair especially at the ends, leave it on overnight, and then the next day, I shampoo and condition my hair. Coconut oil also provides the essential proteins required for nourishing and healing damaged hair.

Weight Loss

Coconut oil is very useful for weight loss. It contains short and medium-chain fatty acids that help in taking off excessive weight. Research suggests that coconut oil helps to reduce abdominal obesity in women. It is also easy to digest and it helps in healthy functioning of the thyroid and endocrine system. Further, it increases the body's metabolic rate by removing stress in the pancreas; hereby burning more energy and helping obese and overweight people lose weight.

Heart Disease

Many people think that coconut oil is not good for heart health because it contains large quantities of saturated fats but in reality it is beneficial for the heart. It contains about 50% lauric acid, which helps in preventing various heart problems like high cholesterol levels and high blood pressure. Coconut oil does not increase LDL levels. LDL cholesterol often makes up the largest amount of cholesterol within the body, and it is referred to as "bad" cholesterol because having high levels of this substance in the body can cause plaque to build up in the arteries and possibly cause a stroke or heart disease. (Stone, "The Difference In HDL Cholesterol Vs LDL Cholesterol")

Coconut oil also reduces the injury to arteries and therefore helps in preventing atherosclerosis. It is also beneficial for pre-menopausal women because studies suggest that intake of coconut oil may help maintain healthy lipid profiles in pre-menopausal women.

Immunity
Coconut oil also strengthen the immune system because it contains antimicrobial lipids, lauric acids, capric acid and caprylic acid, which have antifungal, antibacterial and antiviral properties.

Digestion
When coconut oil is used as cooking oil, it helps to improve the digestive system and thus prevents various stomach and digestion-related problems including irritable bowel syndrome. The saturated fats present in coconut oil have antimicrobial properties and help in dealing with various bacteria, fungi and parasites that can cause indigestion. It also helps in the absorption of nutrients such as vitamins, mineral and amino acids.

Lubricant
It can be use as a natural vaginal lubricant that does not have any side effects.

5. Sun Protection
Sunscreens are products combining several ingredients that prevent the sun's ultraviolet radiation (UV) from reaching the skin. There are two types of radiation UVA and UVB. The chief culprit behind sunburn is UVB, while UVA rays, which penetrate the skin more deeply, are associated with wrinkling, leathering, sagging and other light-induced effects of aging (photoaging). They also exacerbate the carcinogenic effects of UVB rays.

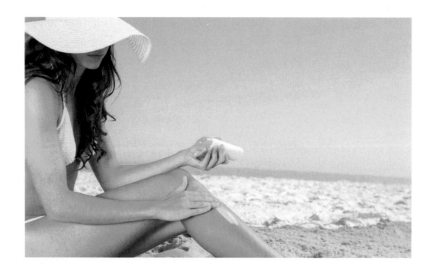

Anyone over the age of 6 months should start using sun protection daily. People who work inside are also exposed to ultraviolet radiation, especially if they work near windows, which generally filter UVB but not UVA rays.

Sunscreens should be applied 30 minutes before sun exposure to allow ingredients to fully bind to the skin. They should be reapplied every two hours and also immediately after swimming, toweling off or sweating a great deal.   If you work outside or spend a lot of time outdoors, you need stronger, water resistant sunscreen. For every day use you can use a light sunscreen that is not sticky and can go well under your make up.   Just make sure they do not contain parabens. ("Sunscreens Explained")

To protect myself against the damage from the sun's rays when they are the strongest, I try to stay out of the sun from 10 am until 3 pm. I always try to play tennis, bike or do any outdoor activity before 10 am or after 3 pm. I always wear a hat, dark glasses and sun protection. (Sun Safety")

6. Whitening Your Teeth with Curcuma

After having been to the dentist for a whitening treatment my teeth ached and became very sensitive. What was more upsetting to me was that after paying a lot of money my teeth faded back to how they were. I felt so uncomfortable that I promised myself I would not go through that torture again. I started researching and found the best method to whiten my teeth naturally:

Mixing 1/8 teaspoon of Turmeric powder and 1 tablespoon of coconut oil.

Instructions:

1. Wet your toothbrush and then dip it into the Turmeric- Coconut oil mix. Brush teeth as normal, but instead of rinsing when you are done, allow the turmeric to sit on your teeth for 3-5 minutes so it can do its magic.

2. Spit and rinse thoroughly, then follow with a second brushing using your regular toothpaste. If you notice any yellow around the corners of your mouth, wash with soap and it will rinse away. If any turmeric powder is left on your teeth or gums it will cause a slight yellow tint, but when the turmeric is fully rinsed away you should notice a brighter, whiter smile. Your toothbrush will be stained yellow after this.

7. Hair Coloring Naturally

I never use to dye my hair, but when I started getting grey hairs, I had to do something about it. I started dying it black to cover my gray hairs, but after my two sisters had breast cancer and I became a Holistic Nutritionist, I did not want to use any chemicals that will be harmful. Standard, non-organic hair dye is loaded with all sorts of questionably safe chemical such as ammonia, formaldehyde, sodium laurel, sulphates and parabens to name a few. In the long run, all these chemicals end up damaging your hair, specially when you have to cover your grey hairs at least once a month.

The organic color system, on the other hand, is a natural ammonia-free solution containing ingredients that are 98-99% naturally derived or organic, and the only synthetic ingredients are the pigments and stabilizers. It has a pleasant smell and the most important thing is that they really work giving the hair a beautiful, healthy shiny color, which does not damage the hair cuticle. To maintain your hair color, avoid products with sulfates and wash your hair less often with water that is not hot. Since I switched to organic hair dyes and organic shampoos and conditioners everybody tells me how beautiful my hair looks. I recommend Naturtint, which does not contain ammonia, resorcinol, parabens, silicones, paraffin, mineral oils, heavy metals, artificial fragrances, SLS, formaldehyde derivatives and comes with its own shampoo and conditioner. I buy them at my favorite natural grocery store Wholefoods.

CHAPTER 8
PRIMARY FOOD

One of the most important things I learned at the Institute of Integrative Nutrition was that the most important nourishing foods for our health are the primary foods. Primary foods are our relationships, the work we do, our physical activity and a spiritual practice that fulfills us.

Many times people use secondary foods to fulfill the lack of satisfactory primary foods. Overweight and disease are the side effects.

You can eat broccoli every day, read labels, eat organic foods, worry about healthy ingredients, but if you are not happy with your relationships, your job or your life you will not feel good, you will not feel happy and it will show.

It is important to have good relationships. Having good Friends is great. Personally, I know a lot of people, but real friends I can say less than 5. It feels good and makes our life easier when we have someone to share our thoughts with, have fun with and someone to lean on when we have a bad day, someone that we can be our true self with.

At this point in my life, I avoid people who are negative, always complaining or like to gossip. These people do not bring anything positive to my life. Some people may think I am selfish by doing this, but at this point in my life, my biggest commodity in life is TIME. I do not want to waste my time with negativity.

After 50, usually our kids are grown ups and have already left for college or got married. 50% of people at this age have been divorced, have married again, and are in relationships or looking for a relationship.

Love after 50 is the best because we really know what we want. We want a partner to have fun with, to take care of each other, help each other, travel together, etc. At this time in our life, we do not want drama or jealousy. We want someone we can trust and be supportive of everything we want to do. Remember, TIME is the biggest commodity we have, as I mentioned before; so have fun and enjoy what you like doing.

This is the time to do something you always wanted to do but never had the time, travel, have sex without having to worry about getting pregnant, meet new people and time to take care of yourself.

I remember someone criticizing me that I like to work too much. For me, my work is not work. It is what I love and enjoy doing. It is my passion. Whenever you feel that you do not like what you do for a living or you do not have a passion for it anymore take the risk and do what you love. Many times people stay in a job that they do not like because they are afraid of making changes or afraid of not been able to make it. When you enjoy doing what you do money will come. I have had clients who had trouble losing weight because they were turning their anxiety and unhappiness to overeating. After they quit the job they did not like, they were able to lose weight.

The other advice is to always keep your mind active. Your brain is like a muscle; if you do not workout with it, it will shrink. Keep active physically and mentally. That is one of the things I really admire from my 90-year-old father. He has been my inspiration in life. He still works managing his business and as a lawyer, edits his own movies, plays the accordion, rides his bike, lift weights, plays golf. He has an amazing memory and sagacity. After 50 he became a lawyer.

Physical Activity

I mentioned already all the benefits of working out and doing a sport or activity that you enjoy. Most of my really good friends and buddies I have met through my love for tennis and biking. By doing the sports I love, I have been able to keep in shape and at the same time met people who share my same interest and live a healthy lifestyle.

And finally, a spiritual practice that fulfill you. It can be practicing the religion you were born with, or a new religion or no religion, meditating, doing yoga, painting or anything that will bring you peace. Personally, I have a small shrine in my house where I sit down for a few minutes everyday. I start by giving thanks for three things in my life, and then meditating. I have found out that through meditation I have been able to be more intuitive, be more positive and peaceful.

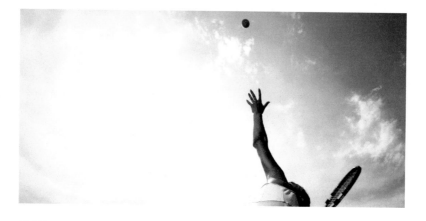

I have always been an avid tennis player and think that life should be taken like tennis:

1. Do not blame others for your faults or problems. In tennis is the same. If you are not playing well do not say that you are not feeling well, or make an excuse. Accept you did not win the match because you did not play well and just practice more and get better.

2. When you are playing tennis and you think too much when returning a ball you will not hit the ball right. The same is in life. Once you made a decision, stay with it and do not have double thoughts.

3. The more you play with a tennis partner that you enjoy playing with, the better and more fun you will have. In life, the more you spend time with you partner or significant other the more you will enjoy life with that person.

4. In tennis you have to be always prepared for the ball to hit it right and be able to get to it on time. The same with life. Be always aware and prepared to be able to catch all the opportunities that sometimes just come once in your lifetime.

YOUR TURN

It is Your Turn to Make a Difference in Your Life

By reading this book, you now have everything you need to start making the changes to look and feel fabulous AFTER 50. If you follow what I say in this book, I promise you will start seeing the changes in your life. You will feel better, have more energy, have less sugar cravings, your skin will look better, and you will have a different attitude towards life.

The candles on your birthday cake are your chronological age but what matters is your biological age, which is the real age of your body. It is up to you to make the little but helpful changes I mentioned. It is up to you to make a difference in the quality of your life. The key is to take action. Make the commitment to yourself to get better and better every day. It is never too late to start.

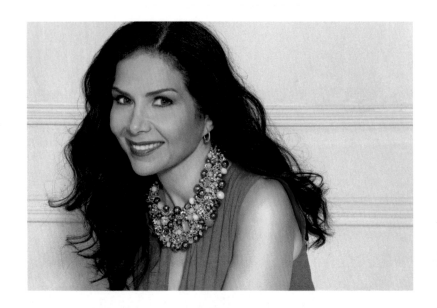

ABOUT THE AUTHOR

Carime Muvdi is a certified Nutritionist from The Institute of Integrative Nutrition and Raw Vegan Chef, who specializes in helping and motivating people achieve their goals through proper nutrition and exercise, creating life-long healthy habits.

She worked as a certified AFFA Personal Trainer and Group Fitness Instructor in Colombia and the United States for 16 years. She had a Fitness TV show, EPS Sports. Carime has presented many health and nutrition seminars worldwide and is the Nutritionist advisor for the Raw Place in the UAE.

She now devotes her time to sharing what she knows with women around the world to help them feel and look fabulous.

THANKS

I want to give thanks to God for all the wonderful opportunities I have had in life to be able to learn everything I know today about health and fitness so I can create a "ripple" effect and share what I know with other people. I want to give special thanks for all the motivation and love I have received from my amazing sons for always telling me "to be up to date." Thanks to my wonderful parents for giving me always the support I needed by giving me wings and freedom to do everything I wanted to do. And last but not least, a special thanks to my father for being my example and inspiration in life.

Thanks to all the people who helped me make this "book-guide" a reality and to all my readers for believing in me.

BIBLIOGRAPHY

Medical News Today. MediLexicon International, n.d. Web. 20 Aug. 2016.

"10 Amazing Benefits Of Matcha Green Tea." *Natural Living Ideas.* N.p., 2013. Web. 20 Aug. 2016.

Ahmed, SH, K. Guillen, and Y. Vandaele. "Sugar Addiction: Pushing the Drug-sugar Analogy to the Limit." National Center for Biotechnology Information. U.S. National Library of Medicine, 16 July 2013. Web. 03 Nov. 2016.

Braverman, David. "Foods to Make your Body Alkaline". Livestrong.com. N.p., 30 Apr. 2015. Web. 25 Aug. 2016.

"Changes in Sperm Parameters of Sex-reversed Female Rainbow Trout during Spawning Season in Relation to Sperm Parameters of Normal Males." Food For Breast Cancer. N.p., 20 Mar. 2012. Web. 03 Nov. 2016.

"Chewing | Mindful Eating Club." N.p., n.d. Web. 24 Aug. 2016.

Ertl, Tunde. "Lymphatic System: The Dust Broom of the Body." Health Secrets. N.p., n.d. Web. 04 Nov. 2016.

"Exercise: 7 Benefits of Regular Physical Activity." Mayo Clinic. N.p., n.d. Web. 04 Nov. 2016.

"Flaxseed: Is Ground Better than Whole?." Nutrition and Healthy Eating. N.p., n.d. Web. 20 Aug. 2016.

Gioffre, Daryl. "Nut Milk Brands: The Good, the Bad, and the Very, Very Ugly - AlkaMind." AlkaMind. N.p., 27 July 2016. Web. 03 Nov. 2016.

"Green Tea Boosts Metabolism, Protects Against Diseases." WebMD. WebMD, 28 Nov. 1999. Web. 25 Aug. 2016.

Grussi, Rachel. "Wake Up Right: Drink Lemon Water | Gaia." Gaia. N.p., n.d. Web. 20 Aug. 2016.

Group, Edward. "7 Benefits of Maca Root for Women." Global Healing Center. N.p., 2014. Web. 20 Aug. 2016.

Group, Edward. "8 Shocking Facts about Bovine Growth Hormone." Global Healing Center. N.p., 24 Nov. 2015. Web. 03 Nov. 2016.

Hamblin, James. "Vegetarians and Their Superior Blood." The Atlantic. Atlantic Media Company, 24 Feb. 2014. Web. 03 Nov. 2016.

Harvey, Philip W. "Parabens, Oestrogenicity, Underarm Cosmetics and Breast Cancer: A Perspective on a Hypothesis." J. Appl. Toxicol. Journal of Applied Toxicology 23.5 (2003): 285-88. Web.

"Health Benefits of Coconut Oil." Organic Facts. N.p., 2015. Web. 25 Aug. 2016.

"Health Benefits of Oatmeal." LIVESTRONG. COM. LIVESTRONG.COM, 2013. Web. 20 Aug. 2016.

"Health Benefits of Salmon | Organic Facts." Organic Facts. N.p., 2008. Web. 20 Aug. 2016.

"Health Risks - Institute for Responsible Technology." Institute for Responsible Technology. N.p., n.d. Web. 18 Aug. 2016.

"Health Secrets Articles - Lymphatic System." Health Secrets Articles - Lymphatic System. N.p., n.d. Web. 25 Aug. 2016.

"How to Boost Your Metabolism With Exercise." WebMD. WebMD, 05 Aug. 2014. Web. 25 Aug. 2016.

"Hydration FAQs." Natural Hydration Council. N.p., n.d. Web. 04 Nov. 2016.

"Is Sugar More Addictive Than Cocaine?" WBUR. N.p., n.d. Web. 18 Aug. 2016.

Bowden, Jonny. "Fructose Turns to Fat Faster Than Any Other Sugar." Jonny Bowden. N.p., 10 Jan. 2011. Web. 25 Aug. 2016.

Lafayette, West. "Study: Artificial Sweetener May Disrupt Body's Ability to Count Calories." Purdue News. N.p., 29 June 2004. Web. 03 Nov. 2016.

Lipman, Frank. "5 Reasons Why You Don't Need to Count Calories Ever Again." Dr Frank Lipman. N.p., 2014. Web. 18 Aug. 2016.

Mcdougall, John. "What Science Says about Link Between Diet and Cancer." Forks Over Knives. N.p., 23 Mar. 2015. Web. 24 Aug. 2016.

Mcnight, Clay. "Does Sugar Turn Into Fat?" LIVESTRONG.COM. LIVESTRONG.COM, 16 Feb. 2014. Web. 24 Aug. 2016.

Mcnight, Clay. "The Side Effects of Artificial Food Coloring." LIVESTRONG.COM. LIVESTRONG.COM, 10 June 2015. Web. 03 Nov. 2016.

"Meissner HO1, Mscisz A, Reich-Bilinska H, Mrozikiewicz P, Bobkiewicz-Kozlowska T, Kedzia B, Lowicka A, Barchia I. Hormone-Balancing Effect of Pre-Gelatinized Organic Maca (Lepidium peruvianum Chacon): (III) Clinical responses of early-postmenopausal women to Maca in double blind, randomized, Placebo-controlled, crossover configuration, outpatient study. www.ncbi.nlm.nih.gov/pubmed/23675006. Int J Biomed Sci. 2006 Dec;2(4):375-94.

"Menopause - Symptoms." NHS Choices. Department of Health, 11 Dec. 2015. Web. 04 Nov. 2016.

"Menopause - Symptoms and Types of Menopause." WebMD. WebMD, n.d. Web. 03 Nov. 2016.

"Michael Pollan Quotes." Good Reads. N.p., n.d. Web. 04 Nov. 2016.

"Michael Pollan's 7 Rules for Eating." WebMD. WebMD, n.d. Web. 20 Aug. 2016. "MSG Side Effects." Healthy Holistic Living. N.p., 08 Apr. 2016. Web. 03 Nov. 2016.

Neporent, Liz. "Out of Control Portion Sizes"." Healthy Living. N.p., n.d. Web. 24 Aug. 2016.

"NHS Choices Home Page." NHS Choices Home Page. N.p., n.d. Web. 20 Aug. 2016.

"Office for Science and Society." Office for Science and Society Does BHT in Food Cause Cancer Comments. N.p., n.d. Web. 18 Aug. 2016.

"Omega-3s: Benefits of Fish Oil, Salmon, Walnuts, & More in Pictures." WebMD. WebMD, n.d. Web. 20 Aug. 2016.

"PCBs in Farmed Salmon." EWG. N.p., 31 July 2003. Web. 03 Nov. 2016.

Pierce, Grant, Delfin Rodriguez-Leyva, and Stephanie Caligiuri. "Systematic Review and Meta-analysis of Flaxseed." The Journal of Nutrition. N.p., 01 Nov. 2015. Web. 04 Nov. 2016.

Pou, Jackie. "The Dirty Dozen and Clean 15 of Produce." PBS. PBS, 2010. Web. 18 Aug. 2016.
Popkin, Barry M., Kristen E. D'Anci, and Irwin H. Rosenberg. "Water, Hydration and Health." NCBI. U.S. National Library of Medicine, Aug. 2010. Web. 04 Nov. 2016.

"Result Filters." National Center for Biotechnology Information. U.S. National Library of Medicine, n.d. Web. 20 Aug. 2016.

Scott, Jennifer. "Top Ten Ways to Control Portions." About.com, 2009. Web. 18 Aug. 2016.

Spencer, Chloe. "5 Reasons to Become a Pescetarian." The Huffington Post. TheHuffingtonPost.com, 29 Sept. 2012. Web. 18 Aug. 2016.

Spritzler, Franziska. "The 16 Best Foods to Control Diabetes." RSS 20. N.p., 17 Aug. 2016. Web. 04 Nov. 2016.

Stone, Sara. "The Difference In HDL Cholesterol Vs LDL Cholesterol." Knowzo. N.p., 30 Aug. 2016. Web. 4 Nov. 2016.

"Study: Sugar Is as Addictive as Cocaine!" ABC13 Houston. N.p., 2015. Web. 18 Aug. 2016.

"Sun Safety." American Skin Association. N.p., n.d. Web. 25 Aug. 2016.

"Sunscreens Explained." Skin Cancer Foundation. N.p., 22 May 2012. Web. 25 Aug. 2016.

"Superfood - Definition of Superfood in English | Oxford Dictionaries." Oxford Dictionaries. Oxford Dictionaries, n.d. Web. 25 Aug. 2016.

Stein, Lisa. "Living with Cancer: Kris Carr's Story." Scientific American. N.p., 15 July 2008. Web. 25 Aug. 2016.

Sutherland, Lee. "Why You Should Start Dry Body Brushing Today." Mindbodygreen. N.p., 6 Mar. 2013. Web. 25 Aug. 2016.

Syuki, Brian. "These 10 Superfoods Can Help Balance Your Hormones and Reduce Inflammation." EcoWatch. N.p., 29 June 2016. Web. 04 Nov. 2016.

Tacon, A.M, "What Are the Side Effects of Parabens?" LIVESTRONG.COM. LIVESTRONG.COM, 18 Jan 2014. Web. 25 Aug. 2016.

"The History of Genetically Modified Foods." Rype Readi Farm Market. N.p., 23 May 2016. Web. 25 Aug. 2016.

"The Truth About Maca." WebMD. WebMD, n.d. Web. 04 Nov. 2016.

Tomberlin, Michael. "Artificial Sweeteners - Toxic Sugar Substitutes." Healthy Life - Healthy Planet. N.p., n.d. Web. 03 Nov. 2016.

"Top 10 Cancer Causing Foods." The Truth About Cancer. N.p., 28 Mar. 2016. Web. 04 Nov. 2016.

"Trans Fat Is Double Trouble for Your Heart Health." Trans Fat: Avoid This Cholesterol Double Whammy. N.p., n.d. Web. 18 Aug. 2016.

"Two Preservatives to Avoid?" Berkeley Wellness. N.p., 1 Feb. 2011. Web. 18 Aug. 2016.

"What Are Primary & Secondary Foods? - Skinny Chef." Skinny Chef. N.p., 2013. Web. 24 Aug. 2016.

"What Are the Benefits of Facial Treatments?" Livestrong.com.Livestrong. com, 2013. Web. 25 Aug. 2016.

Wurtman, RJ. "Brain Serotonin, Carbohydrate-Craving, Obesity and Depression.". N.p., n.d. Web. 20 Aug. 2016.

Zeratsky, Katherine. "What Is MSG? Is It Bad for You?" Mayo Clinic. N.p., n.d. Web. 3 Nov. 2016.

Zivkovic, AM, N. Telis, JB German, and BD Hammock. "Dietary Omega-3 Fatty Acids Aid in the Modulation of Inflammation and Metabolic Health." National Center for Biotechnology Information. U.S. National Library of Medicine, July 2011. Web. 04 Nov. 2016.

BOOKS:

Campbell, T. Colin, and Thomas M. Campbell. *The China Study: The Most Comprehensive Study of Nutrition Ever Conducted and the Startling Implications for Diet, Weight Loss and Long-term Health.* Dallas, TX: BenBella, 2005. Print.

Rosenthal, Joshua. *Integrative Nutrition: Feed Your Hunger for Health and Happiness.* New York, NY: Integrative Nutrition Pub., 2008. Print.

Steinman, David, and R. Michael. Wisner. *Living Healthy in a Toxic World: Simple Steps to Protect You and Your Family from Everyday Chemicals, Poisons, and Pollution.* New York: Berkley Pub. Group, 1996. Print.

Young, Lisa R. *The Portion Teller: Smartsize Your Way to Permanent Weight Loss.* New York: Morgan Road, 2005. Print.

Wignall, Judita. *Going Raw Everything You Need to Start Your Own Raw Food Diet and Lifestyle Revolution at Home.* Beverly, MA: Quarry, 2011. Print

JOURNALS:

Stone M, Ibarra A, Roller M, Zangara A, Stevenson E. A pilot investigation into the effect of maca supplementation on physical activity and sexual desire in sportsmen. (https://www.ncbi.nlm.nih.gov/pubmed/19781622) Journal of Ethnopharmacology. 2009 December 10;126(3):574-6. doi: 10.1016/j.jep.2009.09.012.

MLA formatting by BibMe.org.

37092230R00053

Made in the USA
Middletown, DE
19 November 2016